Healthy and Inforr

CW01589939

Alkaline Vegan Cookery Book

Quick, easy and delicious alkaline plant-based vegan recipes for a healthier and happier life.

Created with love, compassion and peace,

Kimberly Hunter-Gafur, RNCP, ROHP, Registered Nutritional Consulting Practitioner, Registered Orthomolecular Holistic Practitioner, Holistic Nutritionist, Aromatherapist, Veg-Foodie

Reverend Alistair Hunter-Gafur, Personal Trainer, Certified Nutritionist, Metaphysical Minister, Reiki Master, Veg-Foodie

Healthy and Informative Alkaline Vegan Cookery Book

Alkaline: to keep your body in a balanced, healthy state

Cookery: the art or practice of cooking

Vegan: person who does not eat or use animal products

Quick, easy and delicious alkaline plant-based vegan recipes for a healthier and happier life.

About Us

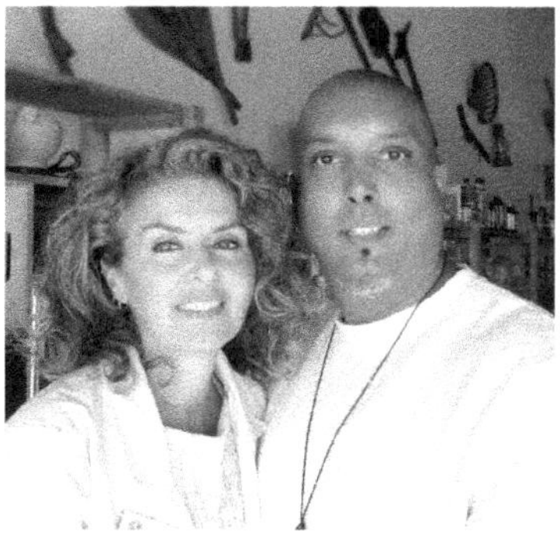

Kimberly Hunter-Gafur, RNCP, ROHP, Registered Nutritional Consulting Practitioner, Registered Orthomolecular Health Practitioner, Nutritionist, Aromatherapist, Natural Healthcare Advisor

Kimberly started her health journey in the late 80's. Kimberly was diagnosed with an auto immune disease which doctors classified as "a black hole in medicine", as they could not figure out what was causing her disorder or how to treat it. After three years and seeing more than a dozen doctors she decided to take her health into her own hands. Kimberly used plant-based diet, detoxification and supplementation to cure herself of her illness. She accomplished in one month what doctors could not do in three years. So excited about what she had learned and wanting to help others, she began her studies to become a Registered Nutritional Consulting Practitioner, a Registered Orthomolecular Health Practitioner and an Aromatherapist.

She has worked for over 30 years in the natural health industry and is currently the proprietor of Alcona Beach Health Shoppe in Innisfil, Ontario. She has consumed a plant-based diet since healing herself more than 30 years ago. Having lived in Italy in the early 80's Kimberly developed a love for cooking. This combination was the inspiration for this book.

Reverend Alistair Hunter-Gafur, PTS, Personal Trainer Specialist, Ordained Metaphysical Minister, Reiki Master, Digestive Care Advisor, Natural Healthcare Advisor

Alistair has always been active and enjoyed working out. Alistair consumed a meat based diet for most of his life and he struggled with acid reflux, digestive and joint issues. In 2003, when he met Kimberly, he began to adapt Kimberly's plant-based diet and instantly began to feel better. He also developed a love for cooking and loves to experiment with new plant-based meals. Alistair also took an interest in Kimberly's healthy lifestyle and passion for natural health.

Alistair is a Personal Trainer, Digestive Care Advisor, an Ordained Metaphysical Minister, a Reiki Master, and Co-Proprietor at Alcona Beach Health Shoppe. He leads all the monthly lectures and seminars at the shoppe and for organizations.

Both Kimberly and Alistair have a passion for helping others. Kimberly has written health columns and recipes for local publications and magazines, including The Globe & Mail. Alistair has written fitness and spiritual healing columns for the same. They provide free public lectures on nutrition, diet and supplementation and are happy to help others whenever possible.

This book is a combination of many wonderful recipes that we have come across, has been shared with us or that we have created keeping health in mind while promoting a healthy, environmentally conscious sustainable lifestyle. We hope that you enjoy this cookery book as much as we have putting it together for you!

We wish you health and happiness always!

Bon Appetit,

Kimberly and Alistair

Index

To Break the Fast

Breakfast *noun*— To break ones fast in the morning, to eat the first meal of the day.

1: Carpe Diem Breakfast Shake
2: Special Breakfast Burrito
3: Middle Eastern Foul
4: Scrambled Tofu
5: Breakfast Berry Bar
6: Everyday Granola

Carpe Diem Breakfast Shake

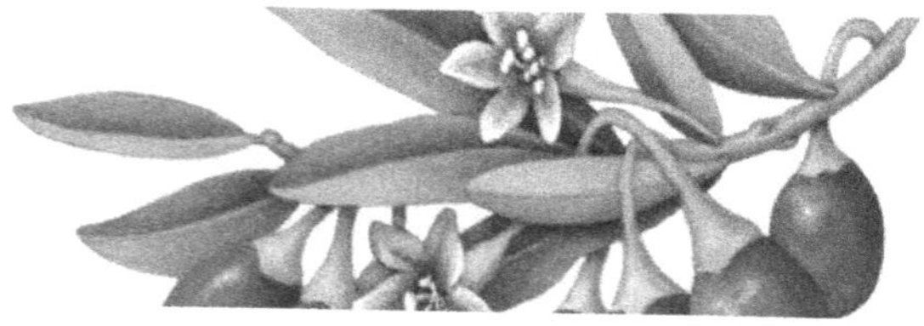

Serves: 2 Prep Time: 5 min

Ingredients

2 tbsp goji berries or 1 tsp goji powder

2 tbsp chia seeds

2 tbsp hemp hearts

1 tbsp mixed seaweeds and algae or spirulina powder

1 tbsp cocoa powder

1 serving/scoop greens complete protein powder

1 serving/scoop berry antioxidant powder

2 tbsp extra virgin coconut oil

1 tsp omega 3 algae oil

2 cups of cold spring water

Instructions

1. Mix everything in a blender
2. Serve in large glass and enjoy the energy!

This power shake will give you energy, six servings of greens, antioxidants, essential fatty acids, proteins, minerals, vitamins, and make you feel satisfied to start your day.

Carpe Diem = Seize the Day!!

The Importance of Breakfast

Breakfast is the most important meal of the day. What you put in your mouth for your first meal of the day will directly impact your mood, your energy levels and brain function. Superfoods such as Goji Berries, Chia Seeds, Hemp Seeds, Cocoa Powder and Coconut Oil will provide all of the nutrients you need to give your body and brain everything it requires to have you function at your best.

Goji *Berries* – Great source of amino acids and minerals such as iron, zinc, selenium and copper. Goji berries are known to help with weight loss, support the immune system and may help prevent age-related macular degeneration,

Chia – Originating from Mexico and Guatemala these amazing little seeds can help to lower cholesterol, help with digestion, stabilize sugar levels, and are a good source of antioxidants.

Coconut Oil – Coconut oil is gaining much popularity. The fatty acids and medium chain triglycerides in coconut oil are known to improve brain function. Coconut oil helps to suppress hunger and increase energy.

Hemp Seeds – High in protein and a good source of Omega 3 and Omega 6. Hemp seed can help stabilize cholesterol levels. Also a good source of amino acids.

Cocoa – Cocoa powder is chocolate in its raw form. It is a powerful antioxidant and this super food will give you lots of energy.

Sea Vegetable Blend –a power blend of essential algae and seaweeds.

Special Breakfast Burrito

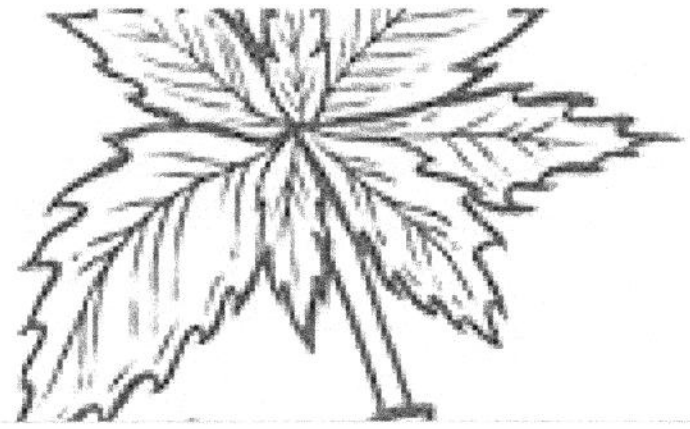

Serves: 4

Prep Time: 15 min

Cook Time: 5-7 min

Instructions

1. Heat the olive oil in a large pot and add the chili powder. Allow the chili powder to simmer in the oil on low heat for about 3 minutes (this will bring out the flavor in the chili powder).
2. Add the soy crumble or tofu crumble, sea salt, black pepper and crushed garlic and water and cook on low/medium heat for about 5 minutes stirring frequently.
3. Place a veggie cheese slice and a quarter of the soy crumble mixture onto each tortilla then top each one with 1 tbsp salsa.
4. Fold both the left and the right sides of the burrito in and tightly roll from the bottom all the way to the top.
5. Place burrito on a hot ungreased frying pan and heat each side until golden brown and serve hot with a refreshing cup of green tea.

   What a great way to start you day. Enjoy!

What Are Soy Crumbles?

Soy crumbles— also referred to as soy ground are simply soy proteins made to resemble ground beef. This is the perfect replacement for any recipe calling for ground beef. High in protein with a fraction of the cholesterol soy crumbles are already cooked therefore only require to be heated up.

Ingredients

2 tbsp olive oil

1 pkg soy crumble (available at health shoppe) or 1 package firm tofu crumbled

2 tbsp chili powder

2 garlic cloves crushed

½ tsp sea salt

½ tsp organic black pepper

¼ cup water

4 veggie cheese slices

4 soft tortillas

4 tbsp organic salsa

Middle Eastern Foul

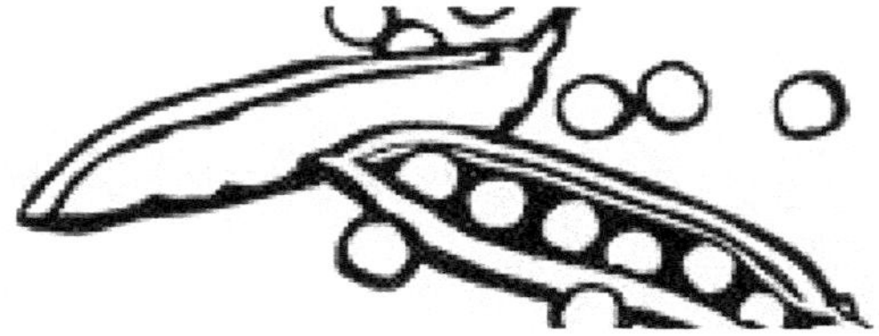

From: Egypt

Serves: 4

Prep Time: 15 min

Cook Time: 15 min

Instructions

1. In saucepan, heat up approximately 2 tbsp of olive oil. Add chili peppers, garlic and cumin. Sautee until slightly brown.
2. Add all of the can of Fava Beans with the cans water and bring to a boil.
3. Turn down to low and mash with a fork or potato masher. Add pinch of salt and ground pepper.
4. Cook on low for approximately 10 minutes. Try it to make sure beans are soft.
5. Turn off heat and add lemon juice and parsley.
6. Serve hot in bowl, swirl olive oil on top. Use warm pita bread or other flat bread to scoop up and enjoy!

The Fava Bean Dish

This is a middle eastern breakfast but also can make a great dip!

Foul, pronounced fool, originated in Egypt but is now a traditional breakfast across the middle east. It can be served with warm flat bread along side of pickled vegetables.

The lemon use in this recipe breaks down bean protein to help prevent gas. This is a good tip to remember when making any bean recipes.

Ingredients

1 can of fava beans (Foul)

2– 3 cloves of garlic, minced

1tsp ground cumin

1/2 tsp chili peppers (or to taste)

olive oil

pinch of Himalayan salt or sea salt

1/2 tsp fresh ground black pepper

1/2 organic lemon

1 tsp dry parsley or 2 sprigs fresh

Scrambled Tofu

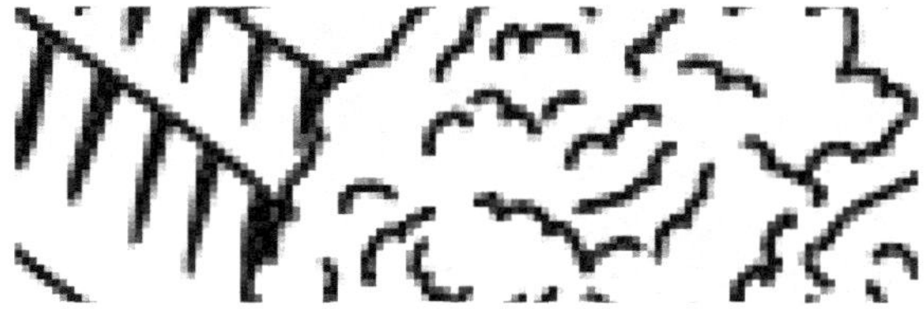

Serves: 4

Prep Time: 5 min

Cook Time: 10 min

Instructions

1. Heat up oil in fry pan
2. Crumble drained tofu into pan, small chunks approximately 1/2 inch. Add soy milk , nutritional yeast, soy bits, turmeric, salt, pepper and mix.
3. Cook until everything is warmed up and the yellow colour is mixed in. Add parsley.
4. Serve with sliced tomatoes.

Healthy for 10,000 years

Soy can be consumed in many forms. Young green soy beans (edamame) are often boiled or steamed and consumed whole. It can be consumed as a milk, yogurt or in solid forms such as tempeh or tofu and in many other formats. Soy has been a staple in Asian diets for over 10,000 years.

Studies have shown that consuming soy may lower bad cholesterol. Soy contains fiber and vitamin K and are a great source of protein.

Ingredients

1 (14-oz) block firm tofu, drained

2 tbsp nutritional yeast

1 tbsp soy bacon bits

2 tbsp Organic oat milk (or any plant milk)

pinch of sea of Himalayan salt

pinch freshly ground pepper

1/4 tsp of ground turmeric

1 tbsp fresh parsley (or dried)

1 tsp olive oil

Breakfast Berry Bar

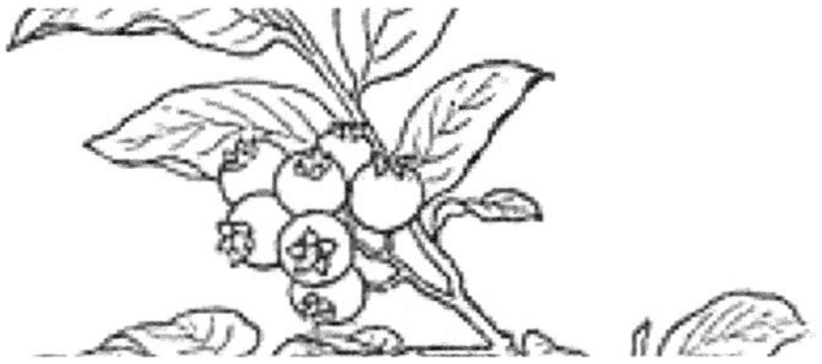

Serves: 4+ Prep Time: 25 min

Instructions

Raw Pastry

1. Grind the nuts, oats, into a fine flour with a food processor or coffee grinder. Place in a bowl and add the rest of the ingredients. Mix together well.
2. Refrigerate or freeze until hard.
3. On a flat surface, flatten the mixture with the palm of your hands or with a roller.
4. Carefully separate the pastry from the surface. Cut into 4"x 4" strips (or any size you prefer) and store in an airtight container in the refrigerator until you're ready to assemble the bars.

Blueberry Jam

1. Place all ingredients in a food processor and process until smooth.

Assembly

1. Place the pastry strips on a flat surface.
2. Top half of each strip with the blueberry jam and fold the other half over to form a sandwich.

Serve immediately and enjoy your day :)

Good Morning :)

This is another energizing way to start the day!

Ingredients

Raw Pastry

1 cup nuts or oats

1/2 tsp sea salt

1/2 tsp vanilla extract (alcohol-free)

1 Tbsp extra-virgin coconut oil

2-3 Tbsp maple syrup, to taste

Blueberry Jam

1 tsp fresh lemon juice

1/4 cup fresh pitted dates (soak dried dates before adding)

1 cup fresh blueberries (other fruit may be used)

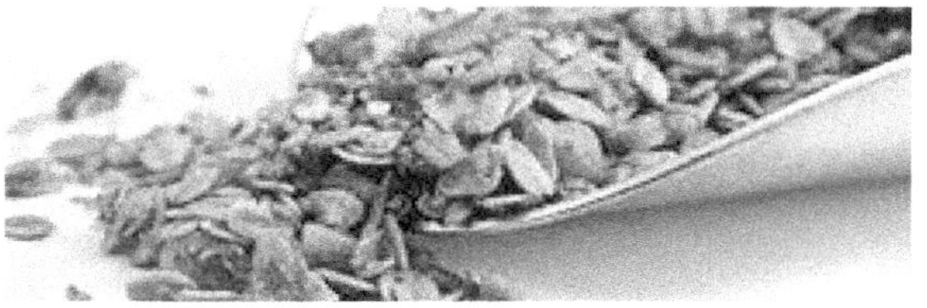

Everyday Granola

Serves: 6+

Prep Time: 15 min

Cook Time: 30 min

Ingredients

½ cups mixed nuts, roughly chopped (almonds, pecans, walnuts, etc.)

1 cup organic rolled oats

½ cup finely ground, blanched almond flour or almond meal

½ tsp ground cinnamon

¼ tsp fine Himalayan salt

¼ cup pure maple syrup

Instructions

Preheat the oven to 325°F. Line a large baking sheet with parchment paper. Set aside for later.

1. Add all ingredients to a large bowl. Using a rubber spatula, fold until clusters form and mixture is well mixed.
2. Pour onto the prepared baking sheet. Using the spatula, gently form granola into an even layer. Separate granola into small piles to create clusters. Make space between clusters to allow for air to flow through and crisp up the granola.
3. Bake for 20 minutes. Using a heatproof spatula, gently flip granola, making sure to keep clusters intact. Bake for an additional 5-15 minutes, until edges are a deep golden brown and granola is just slightly soft. Approximately 30 minutes. Granola will crisp up while cooling.
4. Place baking sheet on a cooling rack. Allow to cool for about 30 minutes, or until completely cooled.
5. Can be stored in sealed container in fridge.

Seize the day :)

Healthy Beverages

beverage *noun*— A liquid suitable for drinking.

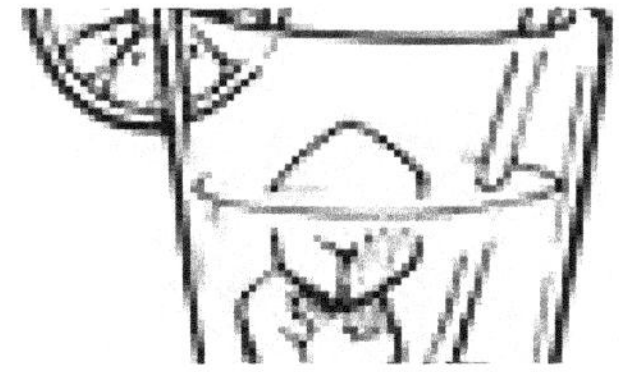

Icy Tea Recipes

Serves: many Prep Time: 15 min

Instructions

1. Bring 4 cups of fresh cold water to a boil.
2. Pour over tea bags and remaining recipe ingredients. Steep for five to 10 minutes.
3. Lightly squeeze tea bags and remove.
4. Add three cups of cold water.
5. Pour over ice in a tall glass, add coconut sugar, stevia or cane sugar. Stir gently.
6. Enjoy!

Healthy Teas

History of tea and its benefits- Legend has it that the origins of tea date back to 2737 BC in the South of China. According to legend while boiling water under a Camellia tree, Emperor Shen Nong noticed that some of the dried leaves of the tree had blown into his boiling water. Intrigued by this interesting aroma, Emperor Shen Nong decided to take a sip and thus tea was discovered.

Tea has since been used for its medicinal properties such as promoting weight loss, lowering cholesterol, regulating sugar levels, antioxidants, promoting better sleep, regulating bowel movements and countless other benefits.

Rooibos Tea — Rooibos Tea, also known as bush tea has many health benefits. Rooibos aids the body in absorption of calcium, improves circulation, contains powerful antioxidants and is caffeine free.

Peppermint Tea— Not only is peppermint tea delicious and refreshing but the menthol in peppermint tea can help reduce stress and act as a muscle relaxant.

Ginger Tea— This powerful root is very popular for reducing nausea, but it also has many other benefits. Ginger can boost your immune system, improves blood circulation and can help reduce stress.

Ingredients

Lemon Ginger with Rosemary

5 ginger tea bags

1 spring fresh rosemary

4 lemon wedges

Minty Fresh Lime

5 peppermint tea bags

1 sprig fresh spearmint

1 tsp lime juice

Black Vanilla

5 organic black tea bags

½ tsp vanilla extract

½ tsp almond extract

Fruity Energizer

5 rooibos tea bags

3 orange slices

Summer Chai

5 green tea chai bags

6 whole cloves

1 cinnamon stick

Simcoe Summer Smoothie

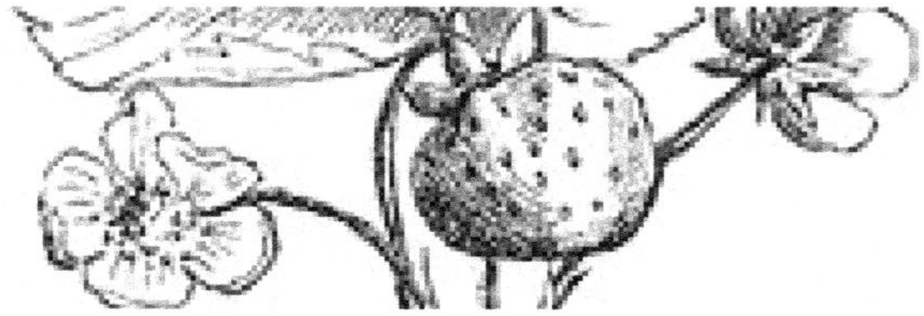

Serves: 2 Prep Time: 10 min

Ingredients

3/4 cup frozen strawberries

1 large frozen banana

1/2 cup chopped cucumber

1 cup of chopped kale

1 cup of spinach

1 cup vanilla oat milk (or other vanilla plant based milk)

1/2 cup of cold green tea (or yerba mate)

Instructions

1. Place all ingredients into a blender, blend until smooth.
2. Serve and enjoy!

Extra Oomph!

Add a scoop of veggie protein powder to this smoothie and it will make an amazing breakfast.

Cheeky Monkey Energy Smoothie

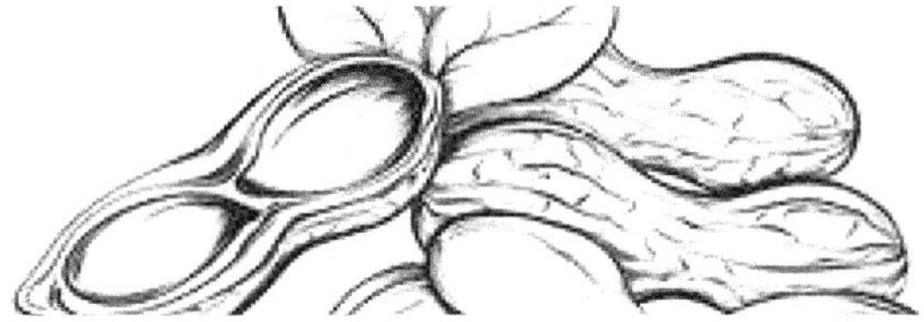

Serves: 2 Prep Time: 10 min

Ingredients

1 tbsp organic peanut butter

1 medium banana

1 cup of oat milk (or any plant milk)

1 tsp cocoa powder

1/2 cup of ice

Instructions

1. Put all ingredients in a blender. Blend until smooth
2. Serve and enjoy.

Extra Oomph!

Add a scoop of veggie protein powder and this is a great after workout smoothie or for anytime you need an energy boost!

Oh Mega Alpha Smoothie

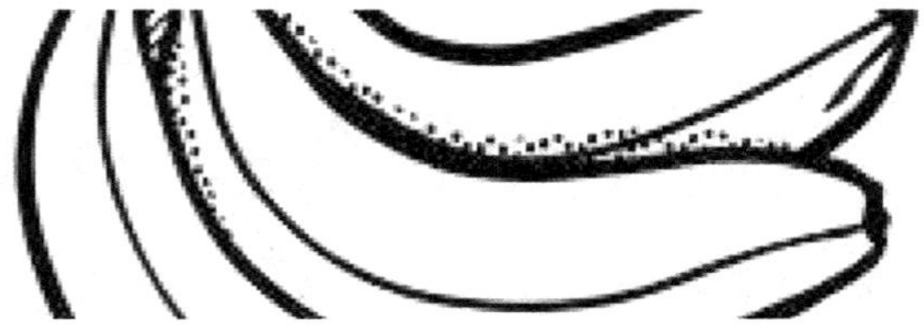

Serves: 2

Prep Time: 10 min

Ingredients

1 cup strawberries

1 medium banana

1/2 tsp cocoa powder

2 dates (pits removed)

2 cups oat milk (or any plant milk)

2 tbsp ground flaxseed

1 tbsp coconut oil

Instructions

1. Add all ingredients into blender, mix until smooth.
2. Serve and enjoy

Extra Oomph!

Add a scoop of veggie protein powder and have as a nutritious breakfast.

Alcona Beach Body Smoothie

PROTEIN

Serves: 2 Prep Time: 10 min

Ingredients

1 scoop of veggie protein powder

2 cups of oat milk

3 tbsp oatmeal

2 tbsp chia seed

2 tbsp hemp seed

1/2 tsp cocoa powder

1 tsp vanilla extract

2 tbsp agave

1/2 cup blueberries

1 tsp maca powder

Instructions

1. Place all ingredients in blender. Mix until smooth.
2. Especially good after a workout!
3. Enjoy anytime.

FYI

Makes a great breakfast too!

Je Suis Canadienne Smoothie

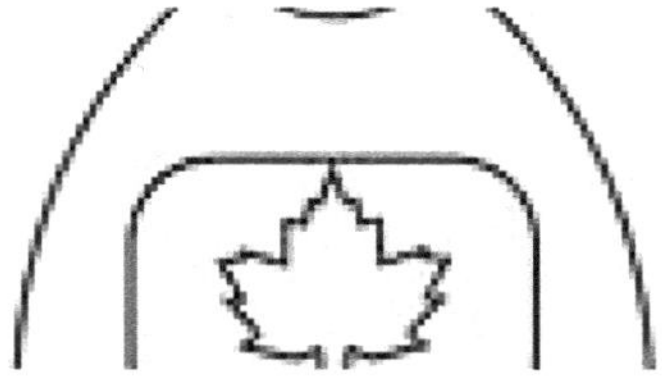

Serves: 2 Prep Time: 10 min

Ingredients

1 medium banana

1 cup oat or coconut yogurt

1 cored and peeled apple

1 tbsp maple syrup

1/2 cup ice cubes

Instructions

1. Place all ingredients in a blender. Blend until smooth.
2. Serve and enjoy!

FYI

Add a scoop of veggie protein powder and this will make a great breakfast.

Sleep-Tight-Good -Night Shake

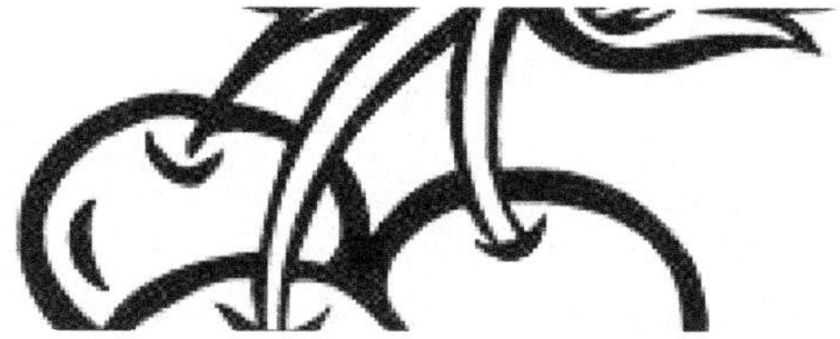

Serves: 1 Prep Time: 5 min

Ingredients

½ cup unsweetened original almond milk

1 tsp organic almond butter

½ banana

5 organic cherries (these can be frozen)

1 tsp organic protein powder

1 pinch of nutmeg

½ cup of spring water

Instructions

1. Put all ingredients in blender until smooth.
2. Drink, enjoy and get a good nights sleep.

These Ingredient Will Help You Relax and Sleep

Bananas – are a good source of B6, which your body uses to make melatonin.

Almond Milk and Almond Butter – Almonds are a source of magnesium which help to promote sleep and muscle relaxation.

Cherries – Cherries contain melatonin which promote a better sleep.

Nutmeg – Nutmeg is high in magnesium which if both calming and relaxing.

Protein Powder – The amino acids found in protein are necessary to create melatonin and serotonin in your body.

Sweet Dreams!

Wintertime Cocoa Drink

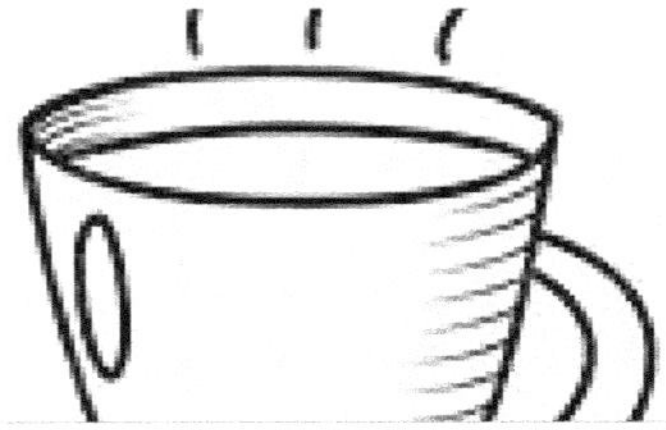

Serves: 2

Prep Time: 5 min

Ingredients

2 cups oat milk (or any plant milk)

3 tbsp raw cacao powder

2 tbsp maple syrup

1 ½ tbsp hemp hearts

1 tsp ground chia seed

1/8 tsp vanilla extract (or ¼ tsp ground vanilla)

Pinch of cinnamon

Pinch of nutmeg

Instructions

1. Blend hemp hearts in ¼ cup of oat milk (with hand blender) until smooth.
2. Add cacao, syrup, chia, vanilla, cinnamon, nutmeg and blend.
3. Add the remaining oat milk to sauce pan and heat on stovetop medium high.
4. Stir in the blended mixture. Heat until desired temperature is reached.
5. Delicious, healthy and full of protein! Serve with a cinnamon stick.
6. Enjoy in front of a fire!

Healthy Hemp Hearts

Hemp hearts which are shelled hemp seeds are becoming increasingly more popular because of their many healthy properties. Hemp hearts are high in protein.

Consuming just one table spoon of hemp hearts can dramatically reduce hunger and improve your digestive functions.

Nog

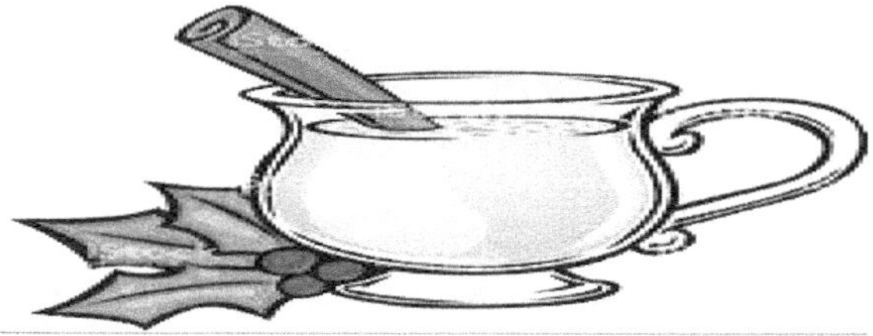

Serves: 4 to 6

Prep Time: 15 min

Fridge overnight

Instructions

1. Combine 2 cups of soy milk and instant pudding in medium sized bowl. Stir until thick.
2. Add remaining 2 cups of soy milk and whipping cream. Mix well and add vanilla, salt and nutmeg and blend well.
3. Refrigerate overnight .
4. Sprinkle with cinnamon and serve.
5. Enjoy!

We be noggin'

Originating in medieval Britain, Nog was originally called posset. Posset was a beverage made of hot milk curdled with wine or ale and spices. Posset was traditionally used by physicians to treat colds and fevers.

Ingredients

4 cups soy milk, oat milk is good too

1 cup non dairy whipping cream

1 oz instant vanilla pudding powder

1 tsp vanilla extract

1/2 tsp salt

1/4 tsp ground nutmeg

1/4 tsp cinnamon

Appeteezers

appetizer *noun* - food or drink used to stimulate the appetite. Usually served before a meal or the main course.

1: Amazing Avocado Teaser

2: Ole Guacamole

3: Simple Traditional Hummus

4: Spicy Chipotle Dip

5: Crudité and Dip

6: Planté

Amazing Avocado Teaser

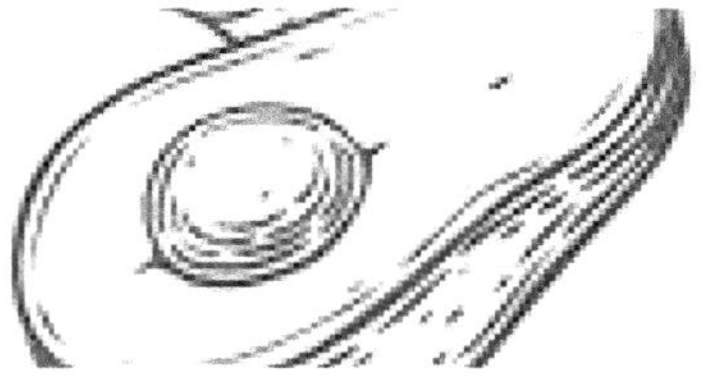

Serves: 4 Prep Time: 10min

Instructions

1. Cut the four avocados in half.

   Helpful Hint: To remove the pit of the avocado once it has been cut in half, use a fairly large knife to chop into the pit wedging the knife into the pit, turn the knife and the pit will pop out with the knife.

2. Place avocado halves into 4 small plates with the skin side down.
3. In a medium sized bowl whisk together the Dijon mustard, wine and dry mustard. The consistency of the dressing should be creamy. If the dressing is too watery add some more Dijon and if to thick add a little more wine.
4. Drizzle some dressing inside the holes of the avocado halves.

   Serve and enjoy!

Amazing Avocados

Avocado- approximately 200 g - 322 Calories, absolutely no cholesterol , vitamin C, potassium, folate, 4 grams of protein, and essential fatty acids.

Don't Throw, Grow!

Open the avocado and remove the pit. Wash pit clean in cold water. Holding the avocado pit with the fat base of the pit at the bottom, insert 3 toothpicks into the body of the avocado about ½ inch deep at the midpoint of the pit (about ½ way up from the base) making sure to spread the three toothpicks a third of the way around the pit.

Rest the 3 toothpicks on the rim of a glass suspending the avocado pit over the mouth of the glass. Fill the glass with water so the bottom half of the pit is submerged in water. Keep near a sunny window and freshen the water daily. Plant in soil when the second set of leaves appear on the stem and enjoy your avocado tree.

Ingredients

Dressing

3 tbsp of Dijon mustard

½ cup of red wine

(we prefer a Shiraz or Cabernet Sauvignon)

½ tsp of Keen's dry mustard

Avocados

4 perfectly ripened avocados

Ole Guacamole

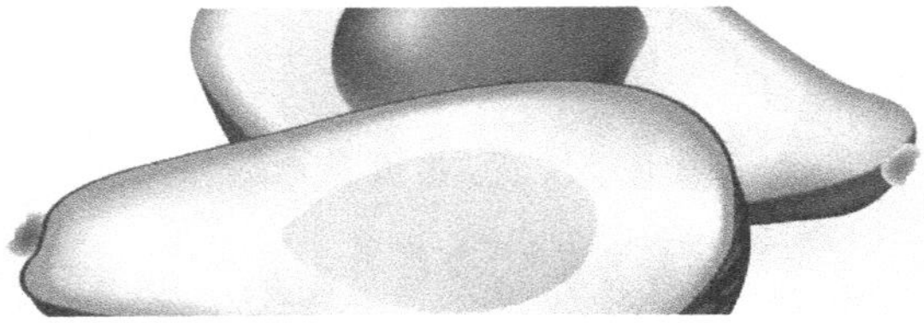

Serves: 4+ Prep Time: 15 min

Instructions

1. Scoop avocados and lemon juice into a large bowl and mash coarsely with a spoon.
2. Gently mix in the onion, tomatoes, jalapeno, salt, pepper and cilantro.
3. Taste and adjust seasoning to your liking, if necessary. Best when served after an hour at room temperature to allow flavours to blend.
4. Serve guacamole with organic tortilla chips.

Cilantro & Jalapeno

Cilantro— Not only will cilantro add an explosion of flavor to your guacamole but did you know that there are many health benefits in this powerful little herb?

Cilantro is anti-bacterial, anti-fungal, an antioxidant, helps with anxiety, sleep and effective for toxic metal cleansing.

Jalapeno— Jalapeno peppers are the little peppers with big flavor but there is an added bonus. Jalapeno peppers are good for you. At only 4 calories each, they are a wise choice for any low carb, low calorie diet. They are also very high in vitamin C, an antioxidant that helps prevent damage from free radicals and Vitamin A which is important for skin and eye health.

Ingredients

2 ripe pitted avocados

½ lemon squeezed

2 tomatoes chopped

½ red onion chopped

½ jalapeno pepper chopped

(more or less to taste)

½ tsp sea salt

½ tsp ground black pepper

½ cup of cilantro chopped (substitute with parsley if you do not like the taste of cilantro, like Alistair)

1 bag organic tortilla chips (or make you own by cutting up pita bread and lightly toasting)

Simple Traditional Hummus

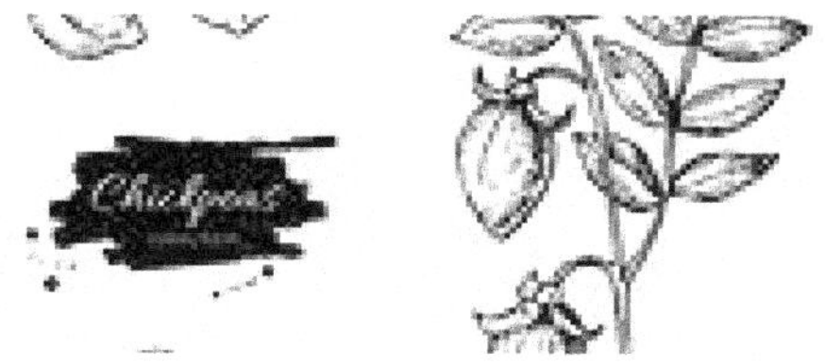

Serves: 4+ Prep Time: 20 min

Ingredients

1 can chickpeas (do not drain)

2 tbsp tahini (sesame butter)

1 tsp sesame oil (optional)

¼ tsp of cumin

½ lemon freshly squeezed

½ tsp salt (or more to taste)

2 tbsp organic olive oil

1-3 cloves of crushed garlic (depending on your taste)

Add hot sauce if you like it spicy!

Instructions

1. Blend all ingredients till smooth, add water to make smoother if necessary.
2. Place in bowl, sprinkle with smoked paprika and a swirl of olive oil.
3. Enjoy with toasted pita bread or whole grain crackers, and veggies.

The Chickpea

Chickpea— Not only are chickpeas (also known as garbanzo beans) high in protein, consuming this yummy little bean will help to lower your cholesterol. Chickpeas are highly effective in the stabilization of blood sugar which helps with appetite control, in turn promoting weight loss.

History of Tahini

Tahini—So what is Tahini? Tahini is a paste made from hulled sesame seeds. This extremely nutritious spread has been used for centuries through Asia, Africa, India and the Middle East is quickly gaining popularity in North America.

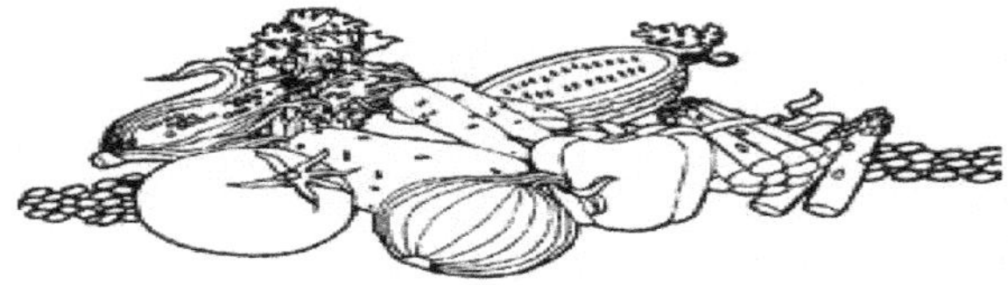

Crudité & Dip

Serves: many

Prep Time: 15 min

Ingredients

1/2 lb carrots washed peeled, cut into quarters approx. 3" long

1/2 lb celery washed and cut in half approx. 3" long

1 red pepper, 1 yellow pepper, cored, washed, sliced 1/2" long

1lb red radishes washed, cut ends cut in half

1lb cherry or grape tomatoes, washed

1 large cucumber, peeled and quartered, cut in 3" length

1 fennel head, ends cut, cut in 1/2" slices

Dip

1 cup Vege-Naise (see Sauces & Dressing)

1/2 tsp dry roasted garlic

1/2 tsp onion powder

1/4 tsp smoked paprika

1/2 tsp dry or fresh chopped parsley

Instructions

1. Arrange all veggies on large platter, keeping each veggie type together.
2. Put small bowl in middle of veggies.
3. mix all ingredient for dip together and place in bowl.
4. Garnish side of platter with fennel leave stalk.
5. Enjoy!

FYI

All veggies can be cut ahead of time and is a quick way to provide snacks for family or unexpected visitors.

Keep veggies cut and ready in the fridge and they will be used as an easy family snack.

Spicy Chipotle Dip

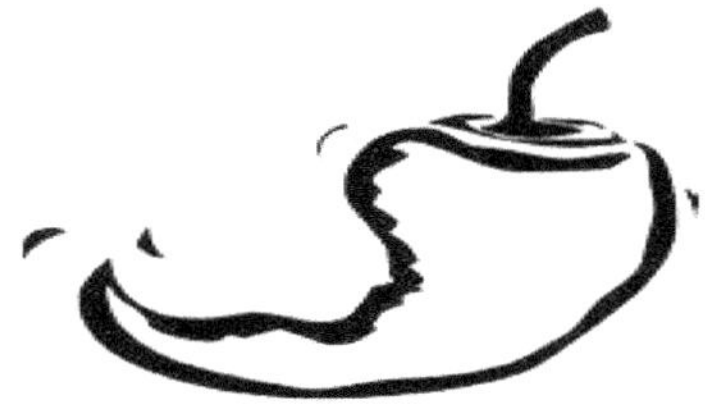

Serves: 4++ Prep Time: 1hr 10 min

Ingredients

1 pack silken tofu

2 whole chipotle peppers in adobo sauce (these peppers are very hot, use more or less peppers to achieve desired heat)

juice from ½ a lemon freshly squeezed

1 tbsp onion powder

3 cloves of garlic

1 tsp salt

Freshly ground pepper to taste

2 tbsp of Dijon mustard

Instructions

1. Place all ingredients into a food processor or blender and blend until smooth (approximately two minutes).
2. Refrigerate for at least one hour to thicken before serving.
3. Serve in a bowl and surround with toasted pita bread or crackers on platter.
4. Enjoy!

(Keep this recipe handy, everyone will ask you for it!)

Protein and your body

Protein is a macronutrient. This means that your body requires large amounts of this type of nutrient in order to function properly. Proteins are used to build, maintain and repair almost every part of your body including muscles, nails, hair, bones and cartilage. Our bodies do not store proteins like it does with other forms of nutrients so it is important that we consume enough protein daily to ensure that our bodies have enough of this vital building block.

Chipotle Peppers

Chipotle peppers are really just Jalapeno peppers that have been allowed to stay on the vine and ripen to a deep red color and begin to dry. They are then smoked for several days. This little pepper is packed full of health benefits including improving digestive function, aiding in respiratory conditions, aiding in weight loss, boosting the immune system and protecting against heart disease.

Planté

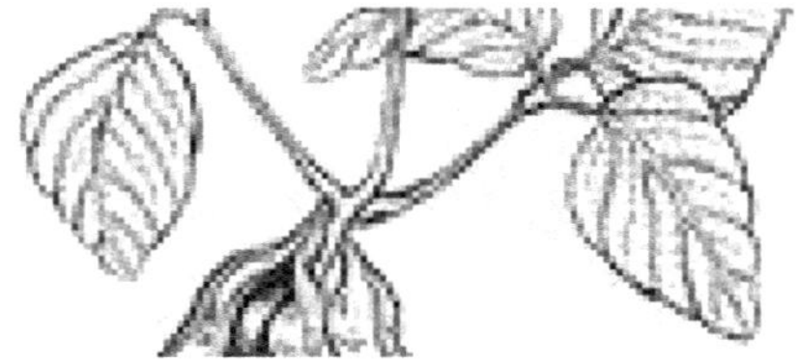

Serves: 8+

Prep Time: 15 min

Cook Time: 20 min

Chill Time: 2 hours

Ingredients

8 oz crumbled tempeh

4 tbsp olive oil

1 cup chopped onion

1-2 minced garlic cloves

8 oz chopped mushrooms

1/2 cup chopped walnuts

2 tbsp soy sauce

3 tbsp red wine

Instructions

1. Sauté the tempeh, onion, celery, and garlic in oil on medium heat. Stir often until onion is clear, approximately 6 minute.
2. Add mushrooms and continue to sauté until tender, approximately 5 minutes. Stir in remaining ingredients and cook over low heat until all liquid has been absorbed. Let cool for up to an hour.
3. Place all of the ingredients in blender and process until you get a smooth brown paste.
4. Spread into decorative bowls, cover and refrigerate for approximately 2 hours.
5. Serve on platter or charcuterie board with veggies, crackers and bread.

This is your plant pate!

Tempeh is a solid block shaped food made from fermented soy beans. Originating in Indonesia, tempeh can be used to replace meat in many dishes. Tempeh can be sliced, crumbled or cut into cubes. It is a very diverse food that can be used in entrees or salads. High in protein and nutrients, the fermented properties of the tempeh promote gut health.

Salad

Salad *noun* [**sal-ad**] a preparation of vegetables usually served with salt, vinegar, oil and spice, and eaten to give a relish to other foods. Leaves that are eaten raw are termed salad.

Easy Bean Salad

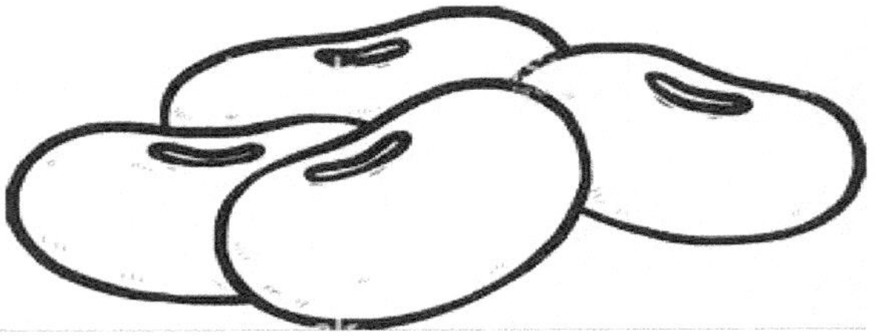

Serves: 4—6 Prep Time: 5 min

Instructions

1. Drain and rinse the canned beans.
2. In a medium sized bowl combine all the beans, celery, red pepper, onion and stir to mix.
3. Add the dressing, salt and pepper and serve.

Ingredients

1 can of mixed beans

3 stalks celery, finely chopped

1 large red bell pepper, finely diced

1/2 medium sweet onion chopped

1/2 to 3/4 cup homemade Italian salad dressing (see Sauces & Dressings)

Sea salt and pepper to taste

Not All Salts Are Created Equal

The differences between table salt and sea salt or Himalayan salt are easily recognizable by their taste and texture. Sea salt/Himalayan is usually coarser than table salt as table salts are heavily processed eliminating much of the mineral content. The 84 minerals and trace minerals contained in sea salt and Himalayan salt add flavor and color making it a preference for many. Table salts also contain additives that prevent clumping.

Greek Salad with Faux Feta

Serves: 4 to 6

Prep Time: overnight & 15 min

Cook Time: 1 min

Instructions

Faux-Feta

1. Bring a pot of water to a boil.
2. Add the tofu to the boiling water and cook for one minute. Remove after one minute and drain. Let cool and divide into 6 pieces.
3. Place the tofu into a glass bowl and cover with 4 cups of water. Add the salt and lemon juice and marinate in the refrigerator overnight.

Salad

1. Put all of the vegetables in a bowl and toss with the herbed vinaigrette.
2. Crumble the tofu faux-feta on top of the salad.
3. Enjoy!

Ingredients

½ pound of tofu

2 tablespoons of sea salt

2 teaspoons of fresh lemon juice

2 small heads of romaine lettuce ripped into bite sized pieces

1 tomato peeled and diced into 1 inch cubes

1 large cucumber peeled and cut into 1 inch cubes

1 medium red onion cut into thin slices

¼ cup of black olives

1 red bell pepper seeded, de-veined and diced

herbed vinaigrette (see Sauces & Dressings)

Onions Are Nothing To Cry About!

Onions— Not only do onions add a flavor explosion to just about any dish but they are good for you too! Onions contain chromium which help to regulate sugar levels and they also promote heart health through the production of HDL which is good cholesterol.

Olive That And More

It is believed that olives were first domesticated in the Mediterranean about 6000 years ago. Olives are an excellent source of Vitamin E. They are a source of dietary fiber and an help to lower cholesterol and regulate blood pressure.

Grilled Romaine with Savory Roasted Garlic Dressing

Serves: 4

Prep Time: 25 min

Cook Time: 30 min

Ingredients

2 small heads of romaine lettuce (one head of lettuce will provide two servings of salad)

1 cup of peeled garlic cloves

1 cup of extra virgin olive oil

¼ cup balsamic vinegar

¼ cup sherry wine vinegar or red wine vinegar

1 tablespoon white miso

2 tablespoons minced fresh thyme or 1 teaspoon dried oregano

A pinch of grated nutmeg

1 teaspoon sea salt

2 teaspoons freshly ground black pepper

Instructions

1. Preheat the oven to 350.
2. Place the peeled garlic cloves in a baking dish and cover the bulbs with the olive oil. Cover the dish with foil and roast for about 25 minutes or until the cloves are golden brown in color. Allow the garlic cloves to cool for about 10 minutes. Once cool, use a spoon to transfer the cloves into a blender. In the blender add ½ cup of water, the vinegars, miso, thyme or oregano, nutmeg, salt and pepper and blend until smooth. Add more water if necessary to achieve a smooth consistency. This dressing can keep covered in the fridge for up to a week.
3. Trying to keep the head of romaine in 1 piece, thoroughly rinse the lettuce. Slice the lettuce down the middle lengthwise and place both halves on a preheated grill or barbeque at medium heat. Grill both sides of both halves lightly (about 1-2 minutes per side or until you can see the char marks). Place each half of the romaine on to individual serving plates and liberally drizzle some of the garlic dressing over top. Serve immediately and enjoy!

Note: the garlic oil remaining in the baking dish can be saved covered and refrigerated for up to a week and can be drizzled over pasta, vegetables, or salad greens.

Garlic, The King Of Herbs

Garlic— This powerful little herb was once used as currency in ancient Egypt and was even buried in the tombs of powerful Pharos. Garlic has many healthy properties include reducing fatigue. Improving heart health and lowering cholesterol. Garlic is an antioxidant and consuming garlic regularly can help remove some heavy metals in the body.

Popcorn Flower Salad

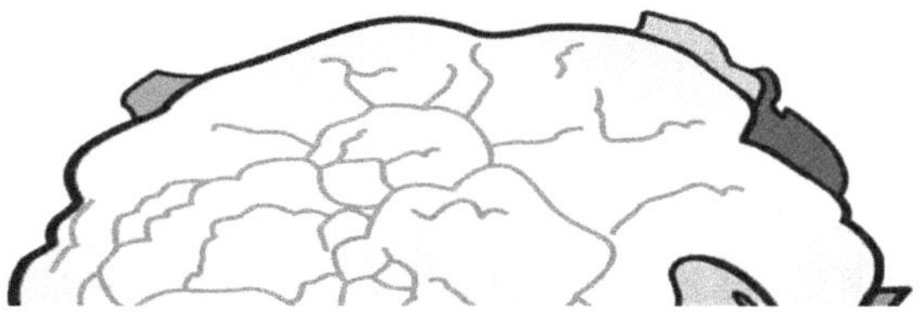

Serves: 6 to 8 Prep Time: 15 min

Ingredients

1 head of cauliflower, washed

4 tbsp of Nutritional Yeast

2 tbsp of organic extra virgin olive oil

½ tsp (or to taste) crushed chili peppers

½ tsp (or to taste) Sea salt

½ tsp (or to taste) Organic fresh ground pepper

2 tbsp Vegasan (see Sauces & Dressings)

Instructions

1. In a large salad bowl put in olive oil.
2. Break up cauliflower head into small pieces the size of popcorn, add to bowl.
3. Sprinkle nutritional yeast, sea salt, and pepper over cauliflower. Mix well.
4. Sprinkle Vegasan on top and serve.
5. Enjoy.

Cauliflower

This member of the cruciferous family of vegetables is unbelievably high in vitamins, mineral, nutrients and antioxidants and boasts a number of health benefits. Cauliflower, and for that matter, all cruciferous vegetables have been found to improve blood pressure and kidney function. Cauliflower is an excellent source of dietary fiber and the indole-3-carbinol or I3C compounds act as an anti-inflammatory. Other benefits include improved heart health, brain health and aids in detoxification.

Seize Her Salad

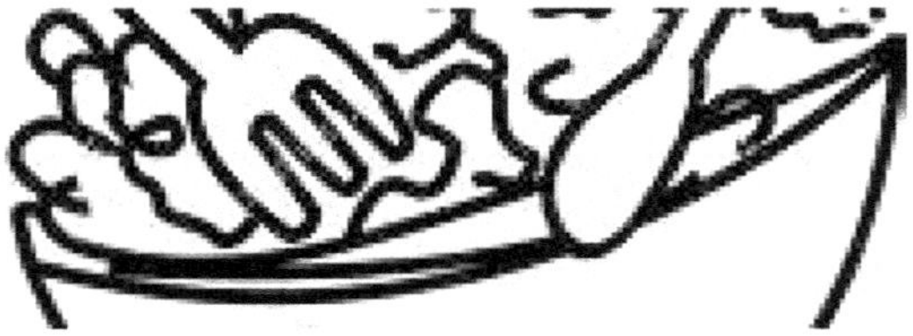

Serves: 4 to 6   Prep Time: 15 min

Ingredients

1 large head of romaine lettuce

½ lemon squeezed

2 tbsp organic olive oil

2-3 cloves crushed garlic

2 tbsp soy bacon bits

2 tbsp nutritional yeast

½ tbsp vegan worstershire sauce

½ cup croutons (optional)

Fresh ground pepper to taste

1 tbsp + Vegasan (see Sauces & Dressings)

Instructions

1. Wash and tear up romaine lettuce into small pieces.
2. In a large bowl mix all ingredients except romaine.
3. When ready to eat, place in romaine and toss.
4. Sprinkle Vegasan on top and serve with lemon wedges.
5. Enjoy!

Nutritional Value Of Seize Her Salad

This Caesar salad incorporates nutritional yeast which is high in B Vitamins, garlic which is has antioxidant and immune system building properties and the organic olive oil provides your essential fatty acids making it one of the healthiest and most nutritious salads you can eat!

Spiced-Up Spinach Salad with Creamy Wasabi Dressing

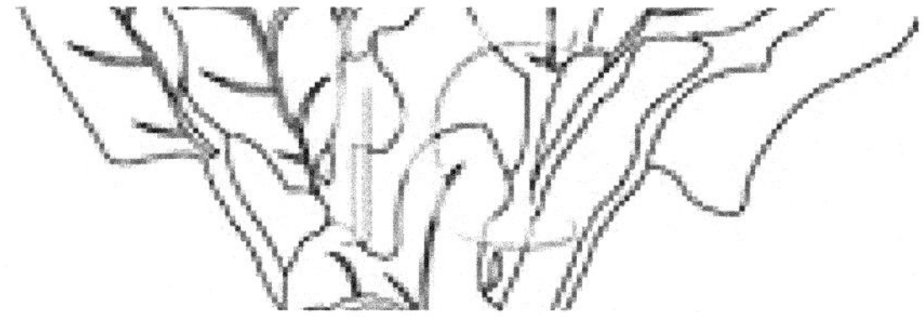

Serves: 4++

Prep Time: 10 min

Cook Time: 2 min

Instructions

1. In a bowl, dissolve wasabi in 2 cups of water.
2. Pour into blender, add Tahini, brown rice vinegar, tamari and blend until smooth.
3. Roast sunflower seeds and sesame seeds in fry pan medium heat for approximately two minutes until slightly brown.
4. In large salad bowl place in spinach, pour seeds overtop and pour desired amount of this delicious, spicy wasabi dressing.
5. Enjoy!

Use for Dips too!

Covered dressing will keep refrigerated for up to two weeks. Also makes a great dip for veg-sushi and veggies.

Ingredients

1/3 cup Wasabi Powder

1 cup Tahini (sesame butter)

1/3 cup brown rice vinegar

1/3 cup Tamari (soy sauce)

1 bag Baby spinach

1/3 cup of mixed sesame seeds and sunflower seeds

Springtime Slaw

(for all the springtime BBQ'ers)

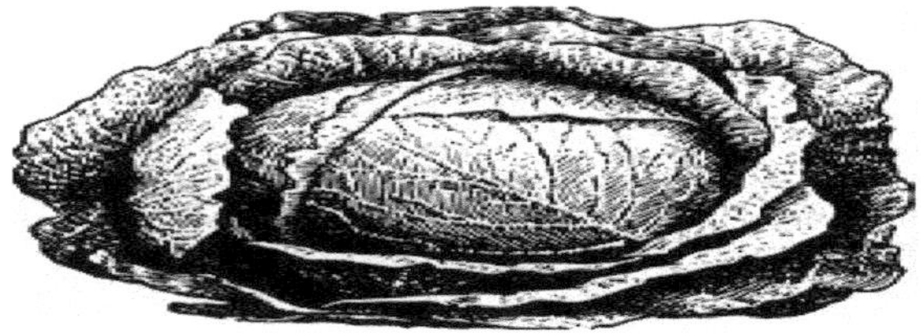

Serves: 4 to 6 Prep Time: 20 min

Ingredients

¼ head of red cabbage - shred

¼ head of green cabbage - shred

1 cup peeled and shredded carrots

¼ cup organic flax seed oil

½ cup of fresh squeezed organic lemon

2 tbsp caraway seeds

1 tsp agave syrup or maple syrup

Sea salt and fresh ground organic pepper to taste

Instructions

1. Toss both shredded cabbages and carrots in a large bowl.
2. In blender mix lemon juice, flax oil, caraway seeds, ¼ of water and syrup until smooth.
3. Strain and add liquid to the cabbage mixture, toss together.
4. Add salt and pepper to taste and toss again.
5. Best served immediately.

What Has More Vitamin C Than An Orange?

Cabbage— That's right, cabbage is richer in Vitamin C than oranges are. Cabbage has anti-inflammatory properties and can help regulate blood sugar.

Tasty Tabouli "Queen of Salads"

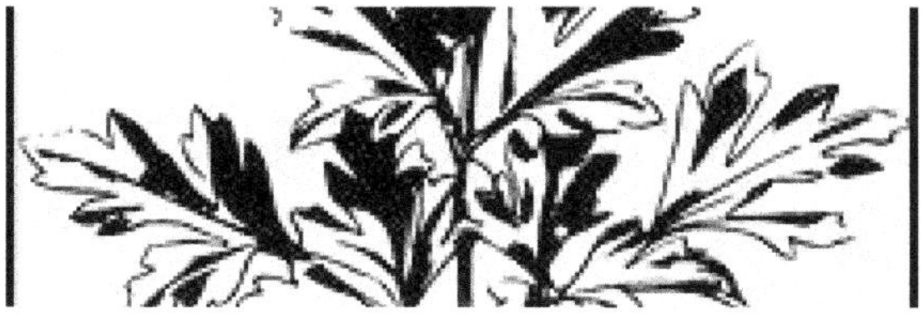

Serves: 4 to 6

Prep Time: 25 min

Cook Time: 20 min

Instructions

1. Cook quinoa according to directions on the packaging.
2. In a medium sized bowl, mix together the tomatoes, onion, garlic, parsley, and lemon juice.
3. Add the quinoa. Add salt and pepper to taste.
4. Serve cool or at room temperature and enjoy!

Tabouli, The Queen Of Salads

Tabouli is a healthy and delicious traditional Middle Eastern salad dish that can be served chilled or at room temperature. This dish is easy to prepare and is and a refreshing alternative to other conventional salads.

Quinoa, A High Protein Ancient Herb

Quinoa contains an impressive 12.5% protein (more than meat) and is an excellent source of vitamins E and C, and contains minerals such as thiamine, riboflavin, phosphorous, and potassium. It also has calcium, making it a good option for the lactose-intolerant. As a source of fiber, it aids digestion. Those watching their cholesterol will be happy to know that it is naturally cholesterol free.

Ingredients

½ cup cooked quinoa

4 tbsp extra-virgin olive oil

½ cup boiling water

2 medium tomatoes, diced

1 small red onion, peeled and diced

2 garlic cloves, minced

1 large bunch of parsley coarsely chopped

2 tbsp fresh lemon juice

Sea Salt to taste

Freshly ground pepper to taste

The Alcona Salad

Serves: 2 to 4 Prep Time: 15 min

Instructions

Dressing

Place all dressing ingredients into a blender and blend on high until smooth and creamy.

Leftover dressing can be stored in a jar in the fridge.

Salad

Toss all ingredients together including dressing and serve in large bowl.

Enjoy your Alcona Salad alone or as a side dish!

Vinegar From Apples?

You may have heard of apple cider vinegar or perhaps it is a staple in your kitchen because of the unique flavor it can add to your favorite recipes, but are you aware of all of the benefits of this powerful liquid?

Apple cider vinegar will aid in balancing your pH level and alkalize your body, increasing energy levels and boosting your immune system while detoxifying your body all at the same time. Apple cider vinegar can also aid with weight loss, and the benefits go on and on.

FYI, next time you have heartburn, take a tablespoon of apple cider vinegar for instant relief.

Ingredients

Salad:

1 cup baby arugula

1 cup baby spinach

½ cup shredded cabbage

½ shredded kale

½ cup cubed avocado

¼ thinly sliced celery

¼ cup ready to eat edamame (out of shell)

1 tbsp chopped pistachios

Dressing:

2 tsp agave nectar

1 tbsp Dijon mustard

1/2 cup olive oil

1/4 cup apple cider vinegar

1/4 tsp sea salt

1 garlic clove minced

black pepper to taste

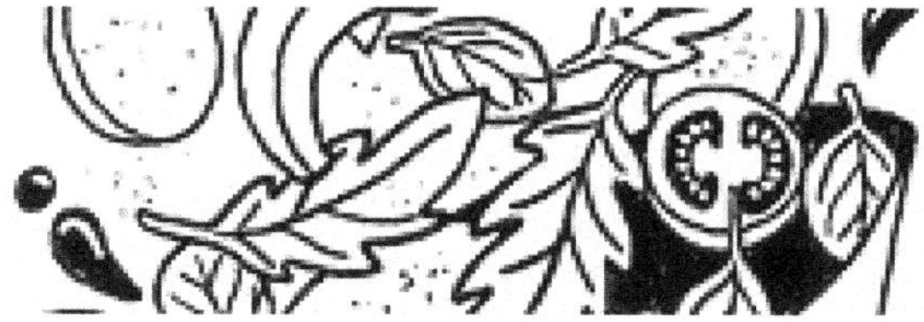

Awesomesalad

Serves: 4++ Prep Time: 10 min

Instructions

1. Break up noodles while still in package. Sauté dry noodles including seasoning package with butter, sesame seeds, sunflower seeds, cashews and garlic. Do not burn. Let cool.
2. Wisk together dressing.
3. Just before serving mix lettuce and noodle mixture together and toss with dressing.
4. Enjoy!

Not All Oils Are Created Equal!

Olive oil, though a little more expensive than vegetable oil, is definitely the healthier choice not to mention better tasting. Olive oils are high in monounsaturated fats which are heart healthy fats that lower LDL (bad cholesterol) and increase HDL (good cholesterol).

Ingredients

Noodle Mixture

1 head Romaine or mixed lettuces

1 package vegetable Ramen Noodles

3 tbsp margarine

¼ sesame seeds

¼ sunflower seeds

¼ cup chopped cashews

1 – 3 cloves crushed garlic

Dressing

¾ cup olive oil

¼ cup coconut sugar (or brown sugar)

2 tbsp Soy Sauce, Braggs Aminos is great

¼ apple cider vinegar or balsamic vinegar

Broccoli & Cauliflower Salad

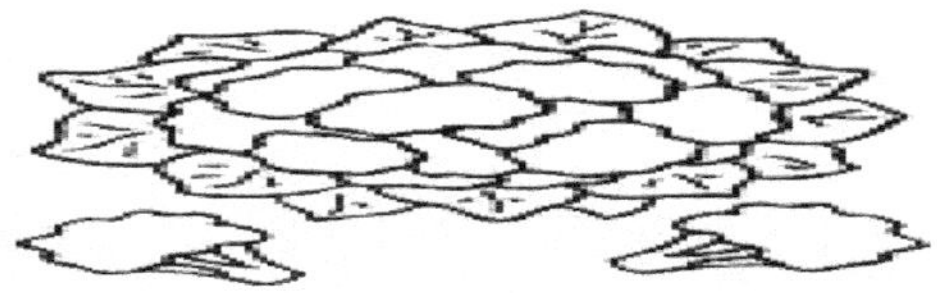

From: mommy Prep Time: 20 min

Serves: 4++

Instructions

1. Mix vegetable salad together. Can be made ahead of time without dressing.
2. Add dressing to salad just before serving. Toss well to coat.
3. Sprinkle paprika on top.
4. Enjoy!

Ingredients

Salad

2 cups broccoli in small pieces

2 cups cauliflower in small pieces

1/2 cup celery chopped

1/4 cup red onion chopped

1 cup frozen peas

1/4 cup shredded carrot

Dressing

1 1/4 Vegan-Naise (see Sauces & Dressings)

2 tbsp coconut sugar (or brown sugar)

1/8 tsp salt

t tsp apple cider vinegar

Soup

soup *noun*—A liquid food of many kinds.

1: Loving Lentil Soup

2: Onion Power Soup

3: Heart Warming Split Pea Soup

4: Energizing Japanese Miso Soup

5: Miso for One

6: Mushroom & Brown Basmati Rice Soup

7: Multi-Grain Veggie Soup

8: Chilled Pea & Mint Soup

9: "What's Up Doc" Carrot Soup

10: Creamshew Tomato Soup

11: Best Borscht Soup

12: Roasted Butternut Squash & Apple Soup

13: Sunchoke Bisque

Loving Lentil Soup

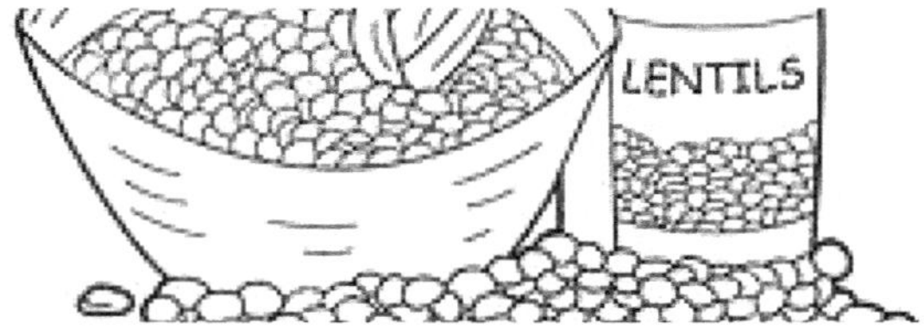

Serves: 6+

Prep Time: 15 min

Cook Time: 45 min

Instructions

1. Fry onions, garlic, cumin and chili pepper until onion turns golden.
2. Pour in lentils, fry for a quick minute.
3. Pour in bouillon water, bring to a boil, then simmer for 45 minutes or until lentils make a creamy consistency.
4. Add parsley and lemon before serving.
5. Enjoy!

For the Love of Lentils

Believed to have originated in the Middle East, lentils are commonly cultivated throughout North Africa, Europe and Asia. Small in size, lentils are a power food. High in protein and fiber while low in calories and fat, they are also an excellent source of complex carbohydrates. Lentils also contain folate, manganese, iron and potassium.

There are 5 varieties of lentils. Brown, yellow, red, green and black (beluga) lentils. Each type of lentil has a slightly different taste and cooking time, but all are packed with nutrients.

Ingredients

2 cups dried green lentils

1 onion chopped

2-3 cloves garlic chopped

¼ tsp of cumin

2 tbsp organic olive oil

Fresh ground pepper to taste

3 cubes vegetable bouillon dissolved in 4 cups of water

1 handful of fresh chopped parsley

¼ tsp dried chili peppers - if you like it spicy!

½ lemon freshly squeezed

Onion-Power Soup

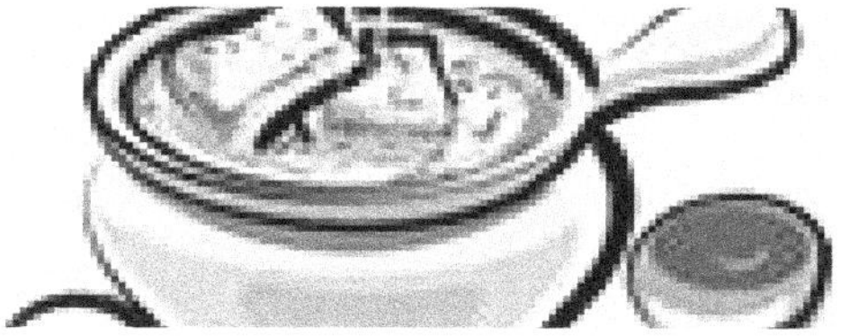

Serves: 6

Prep Time: 15 min

Cook Time: 40 min

Ingredients

2 tbsp extra virgin olive oil

3 large onions, halved and thinly sliced (organic if possible)

4 shallots finely chopped

6 cups vegetable broth (3 organic vegetable bouillons + 6 cups water)

Pinch of dried oregano

Pinch of dried thyme

Fresh ground organic black pepper

2 tbsp tamari soy sauce

2 cups croutons

6 slices of plant cheese

Instructions

1. In large skillet pan heat olive oil and add onions and shallots, sauté until golden (approximately 30 minutes).
2. In a separate soup pot bring vegetable broth to a boil and add the onion shallot mixture, the thyme, oregano, and pepper to taste. Stir in tamari sauce and simmer for 40 minutes. Taste and add sea salt or other seasonings if needed.
3. Ladle soup into six oven-proof bowls, top each with croutons and cheese slice. Put under broil until cheese melts and serve immediately.
4. Healthy and warming, enjoy!

Onion Power

Little is known about the origin of onions. Scientific opinions range from Asia, the Middle East and others believe they were first domesticated in India.

Regardless of where they originated, onions are packed full of nutrients and health benefits. Onions contain potassium, folate, vitamin B6 and vitamin C.

Onions are both an anti-inflammatory and an antioxidant. Onions contain cancer-fighting compounds and promote heart health while lowering blood sugar.

Heart Warming Split Pea Soup

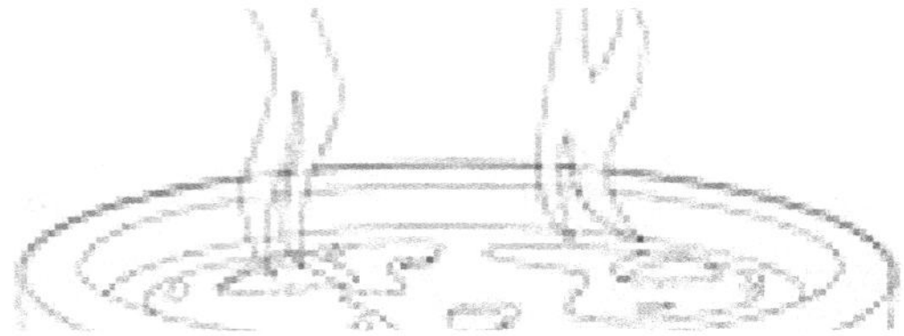

Serves: 6+

Prep Time: 20 min

Cook Time: 60 min

Ingredients

2 ½ cups organic green split peas

1 large organic onion finely chopped

3 cloves organic garlic finely chopped

3 organic carrots finely chopped

2 organic celery stalks finely chopped

Pinch of all – fresh rosemary, fresh thyme, fresh oregano (dried herb can be used too)

3 organic vegetable stock bouillons

1 tsp sea salt

Freshly ground organic black pepper to taste

Instructions

1. In large soup pot, add 6 cups of water with 3 vegetable bouillons, bring to a boil. Add the split peas, onion, carrots, celery and herbs.
2. Stir and bring to boiling point again.
3. Reduce heat to simmer, uncovered, and simmer until everything is tender – approximately 1 hour. Add sea salt and pepper.
4. Serve and enjoy!

Peas & Love

There are two varieties of split peas, green and yellow. Split peas are part of the legume family. Believed to have originated in Ancient Rome or Ancient Greece, split peas have become a popular cooking staple among many cultures used in making soup or an Indian dal.

Split peas are similar to lentils in the health benefits they provide. They promote heart heath and stabilize blood sugar and are full of fiber. They differ in that split peas as they are grown specifically for drying and cook much faster than lentils.

Energizing Japanese Miso Soup

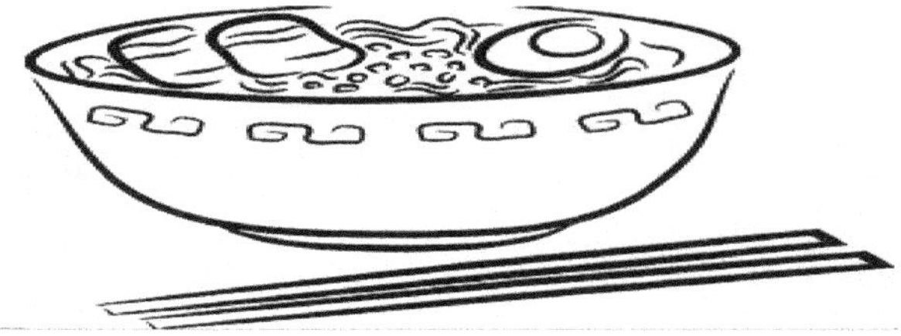

Serves: 4 to 6

Prep Time: 15 min

Cook Time: 10 min

Instructions

1. Sauté the tomatoes in oil and cook until tender.
2. Add bok choy, leeks, and mushrooms and sauté briefly.
3. Add vegetable broth, water, and nori squares and bring to boil.
4. Turn the heat down to medium-low, add the soy sauce and sea salt, and cook for about 10 minutes.
5. Prepare the miso by mixing it together with water and stirring to make a paste. Stir it into the soup—but do not boil. Cook over low heat for another 10 minutes.

Ingredients

2 fresh tomatoes, diced small

1/4 cup sesame oil

1/4 cup peanut oil

1 bunch bok choy, diced

1 large leek, sliced

1 large pkg mushrooms, quartered (shiitake is a good mushroom)

1 qt vegetable broth

3 cups water

3-4 ½" squares dried nori sea vegetable

Braggs soy sauce, to taste

1 tsp sea salt

3 heaping tbsp brown rice miso

Miso Hungry

Miso is a delicious paste made of fermented grains such as rice malt, barley or soybeans. Used mainly in Japanese and Asian cuisine, It can also be enjoyed alone with hot water.

Miso aids in improving digestion, strengthens the immune system, may reduce the risk of certain types of cancers and can aid promoting brain health.

Miso Soup for One

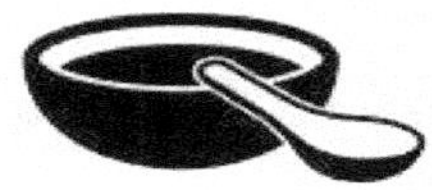 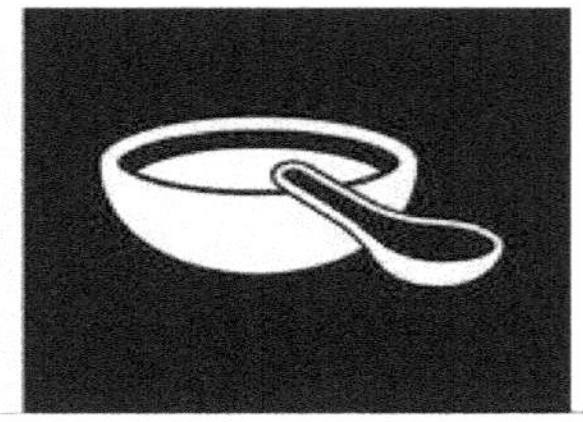

Serves: 1

Prep Time: 5 min

Cook Time: 3 min

Ingredients

1 cup water

3 ½" squares dried nori sea vegetable
1 tbsp brown rice miso paste

1 spring onion, finely sliced,

optional: ¼ cup firm tofu diced small

Instructions

1. Bring one cup of water almost to boil, pour into small soup bowl or mug.
2. Add the miso, chopped spring onions, tofu and nori.
3. Stir and enjoy.

Mushroom & Brown Basmati Rice Soup

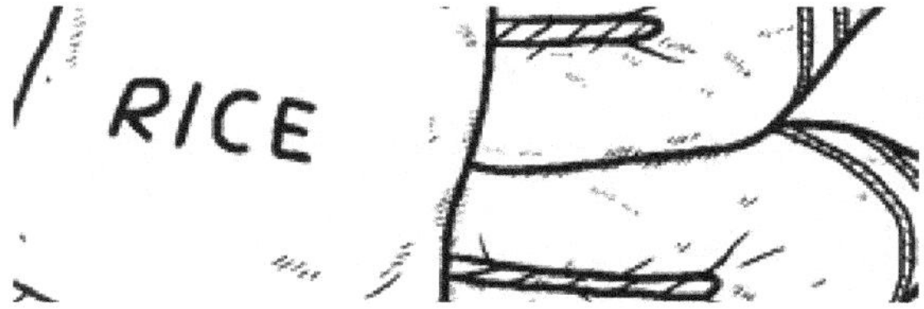

Serves: 4 to 8

Prep Time: 15 min

Cook Time: 55 min

Ingredients

½ cup dry white wine (plus an additional 4 tsp)

4 tsp unbleached flour

2 garlic cloves, minced

1 cup cooked brown Basmati rice

1 small white onion, peeled and diced

4 cups of vegetable broth

½ leek, white part only, rinsed and finely chopped

½ tsp dried oregano

12 large mushrooms, sliced

½ tsp dried thyme

Instructions

1. In a saucepan, heat ½ cup white wine and bring to a simmer on low heat. Add the garlic, onions and leek and simmer for about 10 minutes (until the vegetables are tender).
2. Add the mushrooms, thyme, and oregano and simmer for 3 to 5 minutes, until the mushrooms are just tender. Add the broth and bring to a boil.
3. Reduce the heat and simmer uncovered for an additional 20 minutes.
4. Stir in the cooked basmati rice.
5. In a small bowl, dissolve the flour in the remaining 4 teaspoons of white wine to form a thick paste. Thoroughly stir the paste into the simmering soup and bring to a boil for 30 seconds then remove from heat.
6. Season the soup with pepper to taste.
7. Garnish with fresh time and serve immediately.
8. Enjoy!!!

Beautiful Brown Basmati

Originating in India, brown basmati rice is a unique variety of rice whose health benefits make it a much healthier choice than white rice.

Brown basmati rice is a whole grain, meaning that it contains all parts of the grain. White rice is processed meaning that it has been milled to remove the bran layer and germ. When processing brown rice, only the outer hull is removed leaving the most nutritious parts of grain in tack.

Brown rice is higher in fiber and vitamins and minerals such as iron, magnesium, manganese and B6 to name a few.

Multi-Grain Veggie Soup

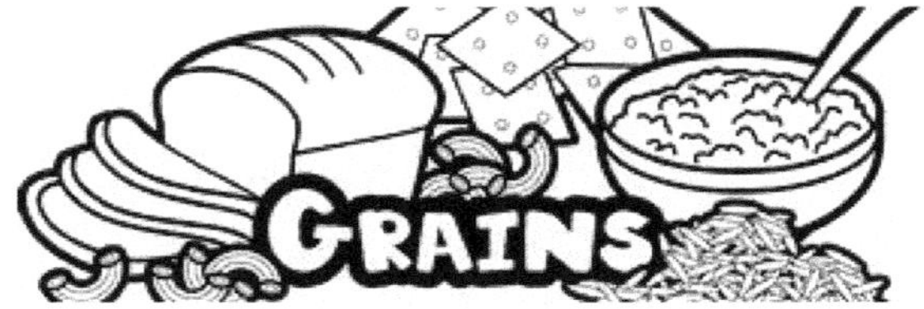

Serves: 6+

Prep Time: 15 min

Cook Time: 1-2 hours

Instructions

1. Heat the oil in a soup pot. Add the onion and sauté over medium heat for approximately 5 minutes.
2. Add the celery, carrots, sweet potato, tomatoes, the four grains, and bay leaves.
3. Stir in the water and bring to a simmer. Add vegetable cubes. Simmer gently, covered, for one hour, stirring every 15 minutes or so.
4. If the soup is too thick add more water and return to a gentle simmer.
5. Add the dill and season to taste with salt and pepper. Simmer gently for another 15 minutes, or until the grains and vegetables are tender.
6. If time allows, let the soup stand off the heat for an hour or two before serving, then heat through as needed.
7. This soup thickens quite a bit as it stands. Add water as needed and adjust the seasonings.

Grain Gains

The term whole grain, refers to grains that have all of the parts of the original kernel such as germ, endosperm and bran. There are many benefits to eating whole grain over refined grains.

Whole grains have been shown to lower blood pressure and cholesterol. The fiber in whole grains promote regular bowel movements. Whole grains contain vitamins such as zinc, magnesium, B vitamins, copper and iron.

Grains belonging to the whole grain family include barley, buckwheat, corn, millet, quinoa, oats, brown rice, rye and spelt, just to name a few.

Ingredients

1 tbsp extra virgin olive oil
1 large onion, quartered and thinly sliced
2 large celery stalks, finely diced
2 medium carrots, peeled and finely diced
1 large sweet potato, peeled and diced
1 28-ounce can organic crushed tomatoes
1/4 cup millet

1/4 cup wild rice
1/4 cup quinoa
1/4 cup pearl or pot barley
2 bay leaves

4 cloves sliced garlic
2 vegetable cubes
6 cups water +
1/4 cup chopped fresh dill

Sea salt and freshly ground pepper to taste

Chilled Pea & Mint Soup

Serves: 4 to 6

Prep Time: 15 min

Cook Time: 25 min

Instructions

1. Heat olive oil in a large saucepan, add the chopped onion and cook for 10 minutes or until the onion is soft but not brown.
2. Add the garlic and cook for a further 3 minutes.
3. Add peas, the chopped mint leaves, vegetable stock. Cover the saucepan with a tight fitting lid and cook on a medium boil for 15 minutes.
4. Blend the soup in a food processor for a thick puree.
5. Return the puree to the pan, season with salt and pepper.
6. Refrigerate until chilled.
7. Serve with crusty, fresh bread.

Summertime Soups

Summer soups are quick and easy especially this Chilled Pea and Mint Soup recipe - fresh summer peas and garden mint are the perfect match.

Ingredients

1 medium red onion, peeled and finely chopped

1-3 garlic clove, peeled and minced

5 cups fresh peas, shelled (or frozen peas)

1 cup mint leaves, roughly chopped

4 cups vegetable stock (4 cups of water with 4 vegetable bouillons)

Sea salt and freshly ground pepper, to taste

"What's up Doc" Carrot Soup

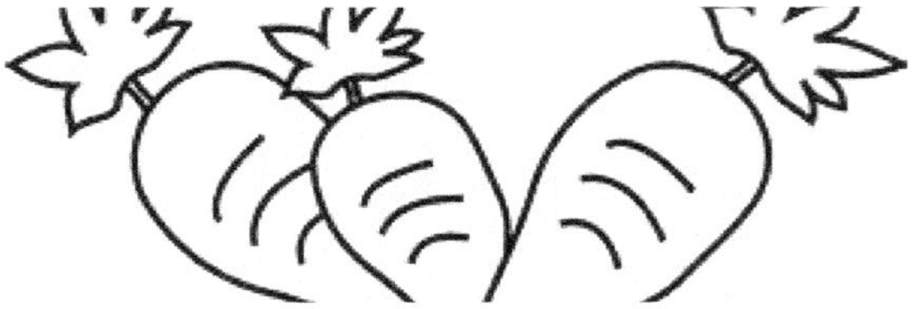

Serves: 4++

Prep Time: 20 min

Cook Time: 40 min

Ingredients

8 cups chopped organic carrots

4 cups diced organic onions

5 tbsp organic extra virgin olive oil

9 cups vegetable stock with 4 vegetable bouillon

2 tbsp nutritional yeast

Sea salt and fresh ground organic black pepper

1/2 cup oat milk to make creamy—optional

1 tbsp maple syrup to make sweet—optional

Instructions

1. Heat oil in a large pot add onions and cook till golden.
2. Add carrots and stock and bring to a boil.
3. Reduce to simmer and cook until carrots are soft.
4. Add salt and pepper to taste and puree with hand blender.
5. Serve with nutritional yeast sprinkled on top.
6. Healthy and delicious – enjoy!

24 Carrot Nutrition

We have all heard that carrots are good for eye health, this is because carrots are rich in vitamin A, however vitamin A is not the only vitamin found in this power packed vegetable. Carrots also contain vitamin K, potassium, biotin and vitamin B6.

Carrots are an antioxidant and may help to reduce the risk of certain types of cancers. They can help regulate blood sugar and may help protect against high blood pressure and heart disease.

Creamshew Tomato Soup

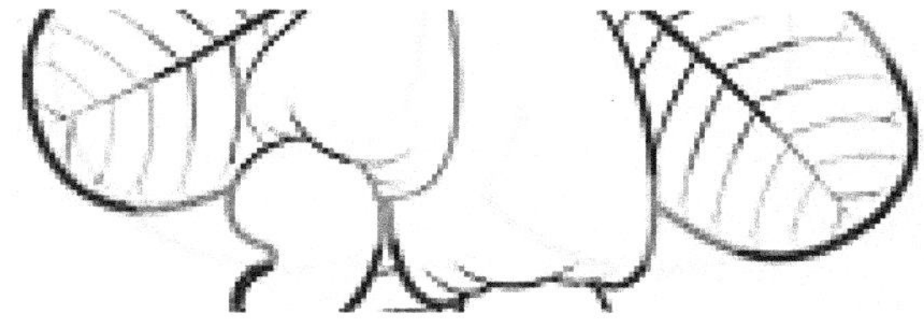

Serves: 4

Prep Time: 20 min

Cook Time: 15 min

Instructions

1. In a food processor, blend together cashews and vegetable broth until smooth.
2. Pour into a separate container and set aside.
3. In a medium sauce pan, over medium heat, melt the margarine. Add the onions and sauté for about 2 to 3 minutes.
4. Add in the garlic and sauté until onions are soft, careful not burn.
5. Add in tomatoes, including any liquid in the can. Reduce the heat and simmer for 10 minutes.
6. Remove from the heat and let cool for a few minutes before pouring into food processor. Blend until smooth.
7. Add nutritional yeast and pulse to combine.
8. Add in the cashew mixture and blend until very smooth.
9. Add salt and pepper to taste.
10. Enjoy!

The Cashew Seed

Cashews are a very unique nut in that they grow very differently than other nuts. Cashews grow at the end or base of a fruit called a cashew apple. They are the only nut solely sold unshelled. This is because between the shell or skin of the cashew and the cashew is an oil that is an irritant which can cause a painful rash. Cashews are not a true nut but more of a seed. They are in the same family as poison-ivy, mangos, poison oak and pepper trees.

Cashews are high in zinc, magnesium, vitamin K, vitamin B6 and vitamin E. Studies show that cashews can aid in lowering cholesterol, lowering blood sugar as well as lower your risk of heart disease.

Ingredients

1/2 cup cashews

1/2 cup vegetable broth

2 tbsp vegetable margarine

1 small chopped onion

2-4 cloves minced garlic

1 28-oz. can whole peeled tomatoes

1/3 cup nutritional yeast

Salt and pepper, to taste

Best Borscht Soup

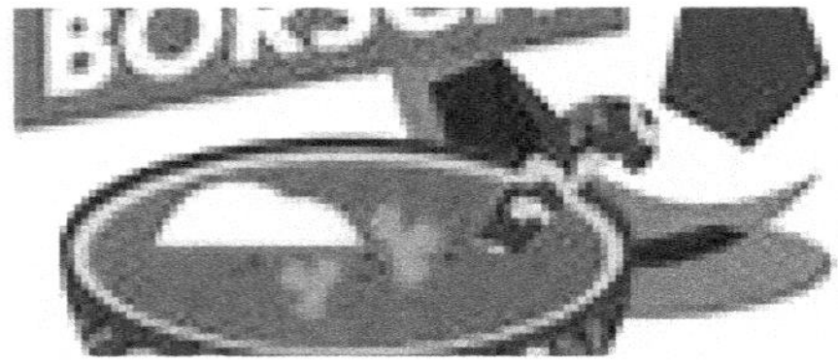

Serves: 6+

Prep Time: 20 min

Cook Time: 1 hour 15

Ingredients

4 tbsp organic olive oil

3 cloves garlic, minced

1 onion, chopped

2 carrots, finely chopped

1 green bell pepper, chopped

3 beets, diced (including beet greens)

1 (16 ounce) can whole peeled tomatoes

1/2 cup canned peeled and diced tomatoes

2 potatoes, quartered

1 cup shredded Swiss chard

2 cups vegetable broth

4 cups water

2 tablespoons dried dill weed

Sea salt and freshly ground black pepper to taste

1 (16 ounce) package silken tofu

Instructions

1. Heat 1 tablespoon of olive oil in a skillet over medium heat. Stir in the garlic and onion; cook and stir until the onion has softened, about 5 minutes. Set aside.
2. Heat the remaining 3 tablespoons of olive oil in a large pot over medium-high heat. Stir in the carrots, bell pepper, beets including the greens, whole tomatoes, diced tomatoes, potatoes, Swiss chard, and the onion mixture.
3. Cook and stir until the chard begins to wilt, about 6 minutes.
4. Add vegetable broth, water, dill weed, and salt and pepper. Bring to a boil, and reduce heat to low.
5. Simmer for 1 hour.
6. Strain half the beets from the broth and place in a blender (blender will be about half full). Hold down the lid of the blender and carefully start the blender, using a few quick pulses to get the beets moving before leaving it on to puree.
7. Add tofu, and continue pureeing until smooth.
8. Stir the beet/tofu mixture back into the pot. Simmer until the mixture is reduced about another hour.

Beet It!

Beetroot, often referred to simply as beets are a power packed root vegetable. Beets are a great source of fiber. They are high in vitamin C, potassium, iron and manganese. Health benefits include lowering blood pressure, supporting brain health, improving athletic performance and improved digestion.

Roasted Butternut Squash & Apple Soup

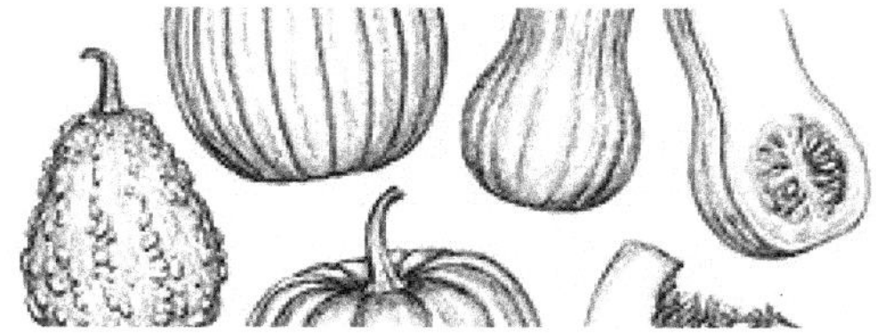

Serves: 4

Prep Time: 20 min

Cook Time: 1 hour

Instructions

1. In a large pan, heat olive oil and sauté the garlic cloves until golden.
2. Add apple and squash.
3. Add salt and pepper and stir.
4. Let cook for 3 minutes.
5. Add vegetable stock and simmer until squash is tender.
6. Blend in pot with hand blender and add maple syrup.
7. Serve with lemon wedges. Enjoy!

Benefits of Butternut Squash

Butternut squash is a vitamin and mineral packed low calorie, low carb vegetable with many health benefits.

Packed full of magnesium, manganese, vitamin A, vitamin C, vitamin E, iron, folate, potassium and more, this vegetable promotes good bone health and digestion, boosts the immune system and there is evidence that it may reduce the risk of heart disease.

Ingredients

1 butternut squash, peeled and cubed

4 garlic cloves, peeled and slightly pressed

2 green apples, peeled and chopped

salt & pepper to taste

2 tbsp organic olive oil

4 cups vegetable stock

1 lemon cut into slices

1 tbsp maple syrup

Sunchoke Bisque

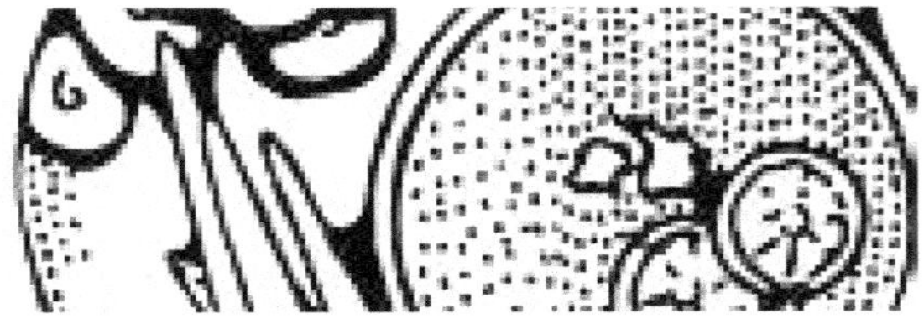

Serves: 4 +

Prep Time: 25 min

Cook Time: 30 min

Ingredients

1/4 cup olive oil

1 pound sunchokes (also called Jerusalem artichokes), scrubbed and chopped

2 small potatoes scrubbed and chopped

1 medium yellow onion, chopped

3 to 5 cloves garlic, chopped

Pinch dried chili flakes

5 cups vegetable stock

1 cup oat milk unsweetened original

2 bay leaves

1/2 tsp cumin powder

1/2 tsp black pepper

Instructions

1. Heat the oil in a large soup pot over high. Add the sunchokes, potatoes, and onion. Sauté about 10 minutes, stirring occasionally.
2. Add the garlic, cumin and optional chili flakes, and continue cooking until the vegetables are lightly browned.
3. Add the vegetable stock, and the bay leaves. Bring the mixture to a boil then lower the heat to low.
4. When soup settles into a simmer, cover and cook until the potatoes and sunchokes are tender, 20 minutes.
5. Add oat milk and simmer for an additional 10 minutes.
6. Use emersion blender for creamy consistency.
7. Enjoy !

Sunchoke the Jerusalem Artichoke

The extremely versatile root vegetable can be prepared many different ways. They can be roasted, boiled, steamed or grilled. They can be cooked whole, sliced, or grated. Native to North America, Sunchoke artichokes also known as Jerusalem artichokes are rich in B vitamins, potassium and iron.

Entrée/ Main

entree *noun* - The dish that comprises the main course of the meal, the principal dish of the meal

Barbecued Polenta with Leeks

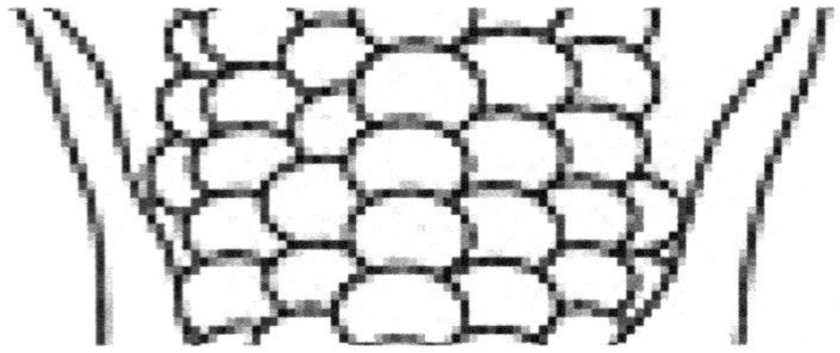

Serves: 2—4

Prep Time: 25 min

Cook Time: 55 min

Ingredients

2 tbsp vegan margarine

3 large organic leeks, cleaned and thinly sliced

1 cup water

2 cups vegetable broth

1 bay leaf

1 cup coarse cornmeal

sea salt and fresh ground organic pepper, to taste

organic olive oil

Instructions

1. Melt 1 tbsp of the margarine in a large saucepan over medium heat. Stir in the leeks. Cook, covered, for 10 minutes, or until softened, stirring occasionally.
2. Add the water, broth, and bay leaf. Bring to a boil. Slowly whisk in the cornmeal.
3. Reduce the heat and cook, stirring often and adding water as needed, for 30 minutes, or until thick.
4. Discard the bay leaf and stir in the remaining 1 tbsp of margarine. Season with the salt and pepper.
5. Brush an 11" (approx.) dish with oil. Spread the polenta in the dish. Cool completely. (Can be made a day ahead. Just cover and chill.)
6. Prepare the barbecue (medium-high heat). Brush the grill with oil. Cut the polenta into 12 squares or triangles. Brush both sides with oil. Place on the grill and cover. Grill until golden brown, about 3 minutes per side. Serve hot.

And the Leek Shall Inherit the Earth

Leeks belong to the same family of vegetables as garlic and onions. These vegetables are called Allium vegetables.

Leeks have many health benefits including aiding in heart health, strengthening bones, aiding in digestion and leeks also have diuretic properties.

Tip

The light green portion of the leek is the edible part of the leek, however the dark leafy green leaves can be used to add some extra flavor to your favorite soup stock.

BBQ Beans and Veggie Wieners

Serves: 2 to 4

Prep Time: overnight soak & 1 hour

Cook Time: 20 min

Instructions

BBQ Sauce

1. Soak peppers in hot water for 15 minutes, drain and pour out liquid.
2. Put peppers and remaining ingredients in a blender and blend until smooth. Taste and adjust seasoning as desired. Add more molasses if you want it sweeter.
3. The sauce will keep in the refrigerator for a week.
4. This is also great for grilling tofu, veggie burgers and on sandwiches!!

Putting it all Together

1. Cover beans with water, add Nori, soak overnight. Rinse and drain.
2. Transfer beans and Nori to a soup pot and cover with two inches of water. Bring to a boil; simmer until tender (approximately 1 hour). Add more water if needed.
3. Drain beans and transfer to large saucepan. Add barbecue sauce and soy dogs, mix well.
4. Cook over medium-low heat until heated.
5. Enjoy!

Make it easier...

If pressed for time you can use canned beans.

Ingredients

1 cup pinto beans rinsed

1 2-inch piece of Nori (yummy seaweed)

1 cup barbecue sauce

2 soy dog wieners cut into 1 inch pieces

Barbecue Sauce

1-2 dried or canned chipotle peppers

1 cup hot water

1 tbsp finely chopped garlic

1 ½ cups tomato paste

1 cup apple cider vinegar

1 cup tamari sauce

½ cup molasses

1 cup agave nectar

¼ cup mustard

2 tsp dried basil

Sea salt and fresh ground pepper to taste

Extremely Easy & Delicious Chili

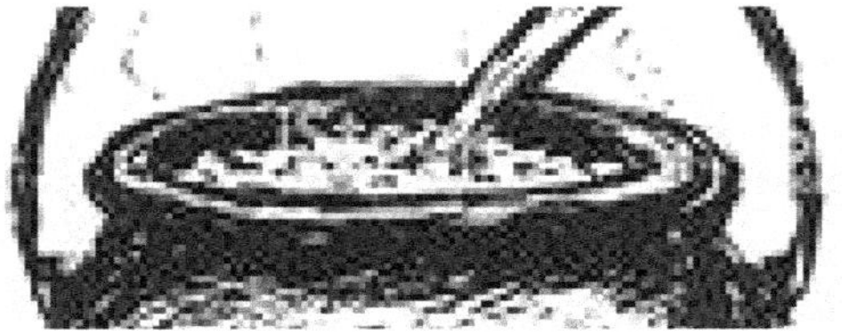

Serves: 4++

Prep Time: 5 min

Cook Time: 25 min

Ingredients

2 cans organic mixed beans

1 can organic crushed tomato

1 package of ground soy

½ tsp cumin

½ hot chili peppers (optional)

½ organic vegan worstershire sauce

½ organic onion chopped

3 cloves organic garlic chopped

2 tbsp of BBQ Sauce

2 tbsp maple syrup

Instructions

1. Fry onions, garlic, chili peppers, and cumin for approximately 5 minutes.
2. Add ground soy and vegan worstershire mix all together for about 2 minutes.
3. Add all other ingredients, mix together. Cook for about 20 minutes on a low heat, covered so all flavours blend.
4. Serve with a slice of wholegrain toast.

For The Love of Lentil Burgers

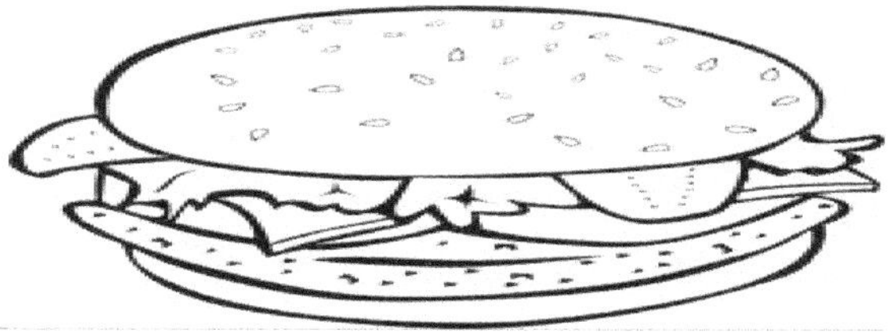

Serves: 4—6

Prep Time: 25 min

Cook Time: 5 min

Ingredients

1 can organic lentils (or one cup of cooked)

1 chopped medium onion

2 chopped garlic cloves

1 cup of breadcrumbs

2 tbsp olive oil

½ tsp sea salt

½ tsp organic black pepper

½ tsp cumin

¼ tsp cayenne

toppings (lettuce, tomato, ketchup or BBQ sauce, etc.)

Instructions

1. Chop up onions and garlic, sauté in 2 tbsp of olive oil.
2. Fry onions and garlic until golden, add spices and mix well.
3. Rinse lentils, then add to onion mixture. breadcrumbs, mix well.
4. Put entire mixture into food processor, mix in food processor until moist enough to form into balls.
5. Scoop portions out and form into patties, approximately 3 tbsp.
6. Barbecue or pan fry, flip gently when browned.
7. Add your favourite burger toppings and serve with a fresh salad.

Grilled Portobello Mushroom with a Red Wine Reduction

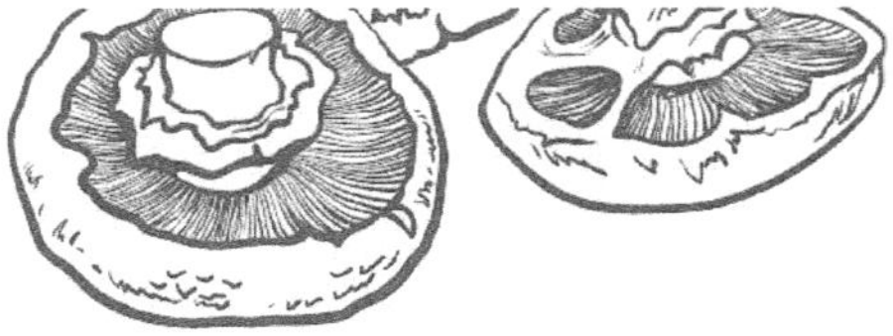

Serves: 6

Prep Time: 30 min

Cook Time: 15—20 min

Ingredients

Marinade

1 cup of aged sherry vinegar

1 cup of olive oil

1 tbsp whole black peppercorn

1 tbsp sea salt

4 fresh thinly sliced bay leaves

6 garlic cloves cut into slivers

5 sprigs of fresh thyme

Mushrooms

6 large Portobello mushrooms

Sea salt and fresh pepper, to taste

Red Wine Reduction

1/2 bottle of red wine (plus one glass for the chef)

2 cloves of garlic, mashed

1 tsp whole black peppercorn

1 sprig of rosemary

1 tart apple, diced small

2 sprigs of fresh thyme

2 tbsp cane sugar

Sea salt to taste

Instructions

1. Remove the gills from the mushroom with a spoon being cautious not to break the cap. Beginning at the edge of the cap, gently peel the skin back towards the center (This will be easy to do once the gills have been removed). Continue until all of the skin has been removed.
2. Soak the mushrooms in the marinade and let sit for 20 minutes and season with salt and pepper while in the marinade.
3. Remove from the marinade and grill for 2-3 minutes per side. Remove from the grill and set aside.
4. Red Wine Reduction—Place all ingredients into a pot and bring to a boil. Reduce to a simmer. Cook until the liquid has reduced to approximately 2/3 the original liquid. Pour slowly over the mushrooms and serve immediately.
5. Enjoy!

Portobellisimo!

Common to Europe and North America, the Portobello Mushroom is one of the more flavored packed varieties of mushrooms making them one of the more popular choices for many recopies.

Portobello mushrooms are the perfect choice as a meat replacement because of their flavor and texture and their ability to absorb the flavor of any marinade or seasoning used on them.

Portobello Mushrooms are a great source of protein. They are low in saturated fats and sodium but high in other important vitamins and minerals such as Zinc, Magnesium, Manganese, Vitamin B6, Potassium and much more.

These mushrooms are a natural anti-inflammatory and a great source of antioxidants.

Authentic Herbed Risotto

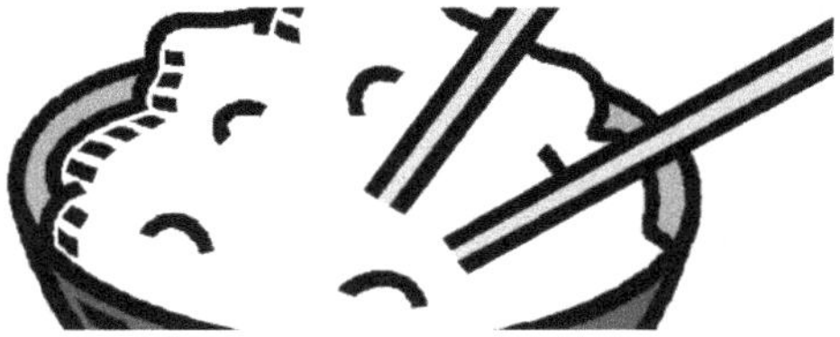

Straight from Italia

Prep Time: 45 min

Serves: 4

Cook Time: 20-25 min

Ingredients

½ cup dry white wine

4 cups of vegetable bouillon broth (1 vegetable bouillon per cup of water)

2 tablespoons organic olive oil

2-4 cloves of garlic minced

1/2 large onion diced

4 tablespoons of nutritional yeast

2 cups Arborio rice

¼ tsp of each – dried oregano, dried thyme, basil

1 tbsp dried parsley

Freshly ground black pepper to taste

¼ tsp chili peppers (optional)

Instructions

1. In a saucepan, bring vegetable bouillon broth to a boil, and then simmer over very low heat.
2. In a large soup pot over medium heat, add olive oil. Add the onions and garlic until golden.
3. Add all herbs, and rice and stir until well coated.
4. Add wine. Sautee for 1 minute. Add ½ a cup of the simmering broth and bring to a boil. Reduce the heat and simmer gently while stirring frequently until most of the liquid is absorbed.
5. Continue to add the liquid in ½ cup at a time and stir until the rice has absorbed all of it. This will take about 20-25 minutes. The rice is done when it is creamy and not soupy. The rice will be tender but not mushy and will still retain its bite. (Add more water if needed)
6. Add in nutritional yeast and stir well.
7. Divide the risotto into 4 large pasta bowls and sprinkle a little nutritional yeast, fresh ground pepper - serve immediately.
8. Buon Appetito!

Arborio Rice

The secret to perfect, creamy risotto is to use the right type of rice and to stir the broth constantly while the rice is simmering.

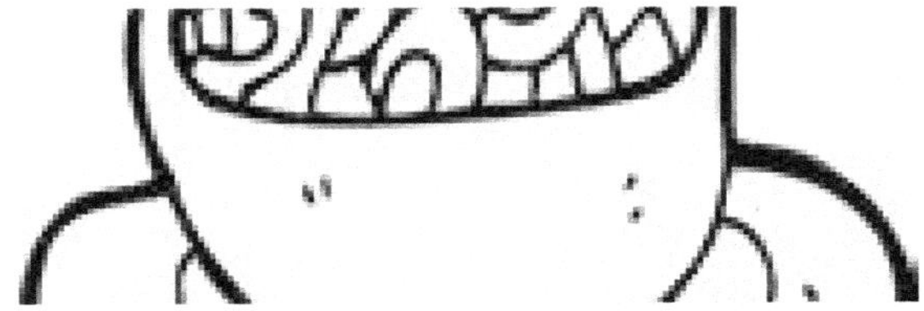

Macincheeze

Serves: 4++

Prep Time: 25 min

Cook Time: 25 min

Instructions

1. Combine the flour, nutritional yeast, chili powder, salt and garlic powder in saucepan.
2. Then add the hot water slowly, whisking constantly. Warm the mixture over medium heat, stirring often and taking care not to burn it.
3. Add the oil, mustard and vinegar. Continue cooking and stirring the mixture until thick. Add extra salt, garlic or chili powder to taste.
4. In a large pot, cook the pasta according to the package instructions.
5. Drain and mix in the cheeze sauce. Sprinkle a little nutritional yeast and fresh ground pepper on top.
6. Enjoy!!

Ingredients

Cheeze

2 cups white flour

2 cups Nutritional Yeast (available at health stores)

2 tsp chili powder

1 tbsp fine sea salt

1 tbsp garlic powder

8 cups hot water

1 cup safflower oil

2 tbsp prepared mustard

2 tbsp apple cider vinegar

Mac

4 cups macaroni pasta (other pasta can be used too)

Lasagna they will come back for!

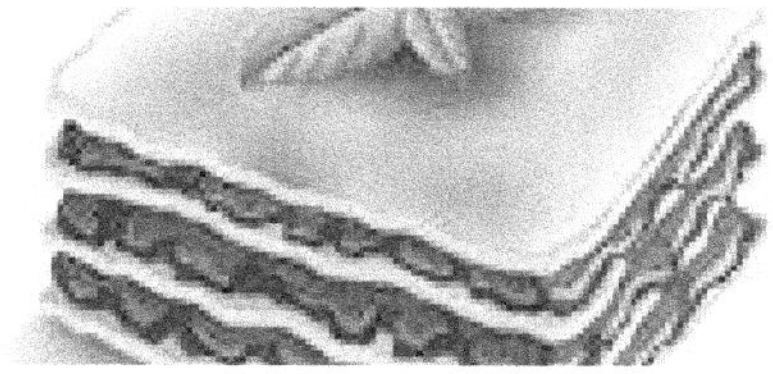

Serves: 6++

Prep Time: 25 min

Cook Time: 35 min

Instructions

1. Cook 9 pieces of brown rice lasagna pasta. Cook about 3 minutes less than on package instructions. Rinse.
2. In the bottom of lasagna dish (low rectangular approximately 12" Pyrex or ceramic dish) rub olive oil to slightly cover bottom of dish.
3. Add a thin layer of the MTM.
4. Place 3 lasagna beside each other. Then layer 1/3 of the MTM. Layer ½ the Tofu Ricotta.
5. Repeat pasta, MTM, Ricotta layering.
6. End with the last 3 lasagna and MTM on top.
7. Sprinkle a thin layer of nutritional yeast on top and some fresh ground pepper.
8. Cover with tin foil.
9. Cook for 35 minutes at 350°.
10. Let cool down about 5 minutes to set and enjoy!

Nutritional Yeast

Nutritional Yeast is found in health stores. It has a delicious taste, full of B-complex for energy and chromium to regulate sugar/glucose levels – use anytime you would use parmesan or cheese.

Brown rice pasta is gluten-free, easier to digest, does not break down to sugar as fast as wheat pasta, and has more taste.

Ingredients

Tofu Ricotta

1 pound firm tofu

1 tsp dried basil

1 tsp dried thyme

1 tsp dried oregano

2 tsp sea salt

½ tsp freshly ground black pepper

Combine all these ingredients in a food processor until fine consistency. Add water if needed.

"Meaty" Tomato Sauce MTM

2 28 oz can of crushed tomatoes

1 package of ground soy (substitute with can of beans)

1 tsp dried basil

Chili peppers to taste

3 cloves garlic – crushed

1 onion finely chopped

Fry onions, garlic till slightly golden, add ground soy, cook for less than one minute, add crushed tomatoes and remaining ingredients.

Topping

Approx. 2 tbsp Nutritional Yeast

Artichoke Pesto Pasta

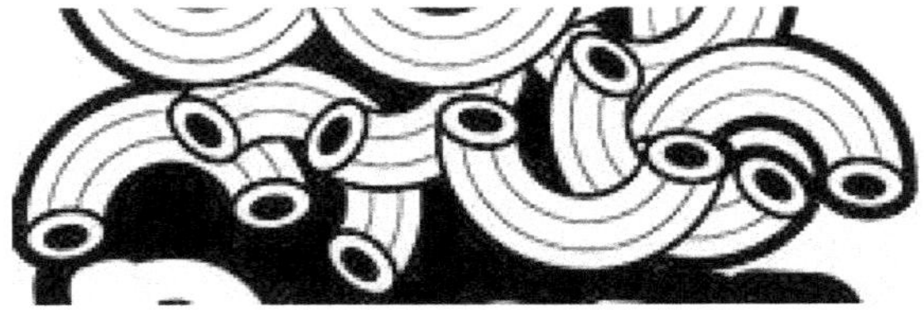

Serves: 4 to 6

Prep Time: 10 min

Cook Time: 15 min

Ingredients

2 cups rice pasta (penne is good)

1 chopped large tomato

1 170ml jar marinated artichoke hearts – drained and chopped

1/3 cup lightly toasted pine nuts

2-4 crushed garlic cloves

¼ cup finely chopped fresh basil

¼ tsp dried oregano

2 tbsp organic olive oil

½ tsp freshly ground black pepper (or to taste)

¼ tsp sea salt

Instructions

In large pasta pot, boil salted water and cook pasta. (Hint: When cooking rice pastas, taste it a couple minutes before the suggested cooking time to see if it is to your liking)

While pasta is cooking place pine nuts, garlic and olive oil in large sauce pan and sauté on medium heat until softened. Add tomatoes, artichoke, basil, oregano, pepper and salt, stir till heated.

Drain pasta, rinse and return the pasta to the pot. Add artichoke mixture, toss well. Serve in big pasta bowls. Enjoy with a fresh, crisp salad.

Pining for Nuts

Pine nuts are cultivated from the pine stone which come from, of course, the pine tree. However, there are only about 20 species of pine trees that produce edible pine nuts. Growing and harvesting these nuts from their protective cone takes a great deal of time. This is why pine nuts are one of the more expensive nuts in grocery stores. However, they are worth the price.

Not only are they packed full of flavor, but they boast many health benefits including aiding in the prevention of heart disease, preventing eye disease, they promote bone heath and they feed the brain.

Lemon Herb Baked Tofu

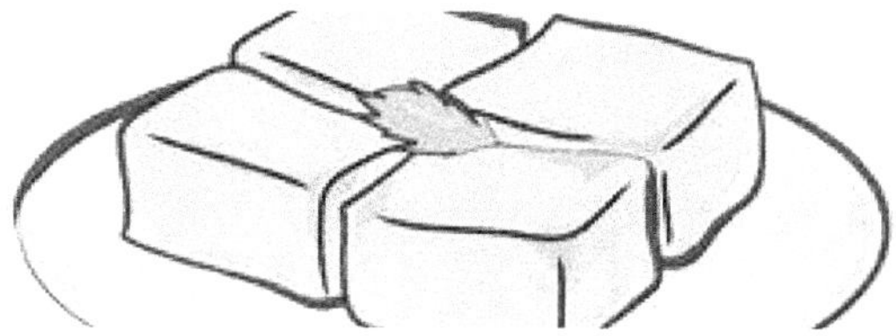

Serves: 4—6

Prep Time: 10 min

Cook Time: 35 min

Ingredients

1 lb extra firm organic tofu

(sliced lengthwise into three)

1 whole lemon squeezed

2 tbsp organic olive oil

2 tbsp organic soy sauce

2 tbsp chopped (or ½ tsp dried) thyme

Note: this is a great dish for tofu first-timers, cook it well and everyone will love it!

Instructions

1. Place sliced tofu in baking dish.
2. Pour mixed ingredient over all tofu and turn tofu over once to coat.
3. Marinate all day, if possible (make this in the morning and pop in the oven when you are ready for dinner).
4. Bake at 475 degrees for 35 minutes turning over once half way through baking.
5. Serve on a bed of brown basmati rice.
6. Enjoy!

Pressing Tofu Matters

Pressing excess moisture out of your tofu makes it firmer and thirsty, meaning that it is better able to absorb marinades. This works best with extra firm tofu.

Pressing your tofu is very easy. Remove the tofu from its packaging and drain. Then simply wrap your tofu in a dish cloth or paper towels and rest it on a cookie sheet or cutting board.

Place another flat object such as a plate or cutting board on top of the wrapped tofu and place something to use as a weight on top of the whatever the flat object you are using (A few cans will do the trick—such as canned beans or tomatoes).

Let sit for an hour or longer if possible. If the tofu is exceptionally wet then you may want to change the dish towel or paper towels after about a half an hour. :)

Ola Nachos

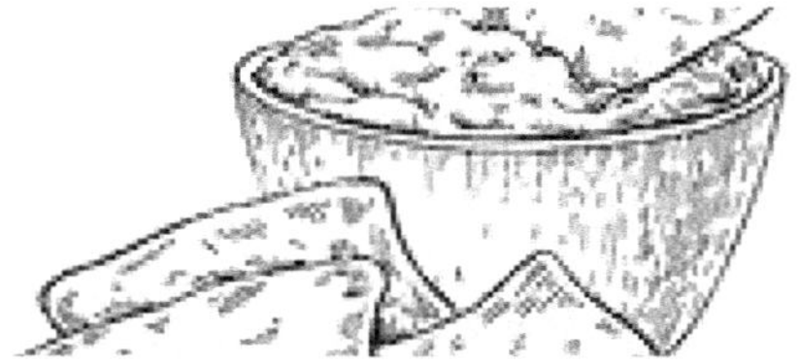

Serves: 4—6

Prep Time: 15 min

Cook Time: 5-10 min

Instructions

1. Preheat the oven to 350 F.
2. On a large baking sheet, spread out a single layer of tortillas covering the baking sheet.
3. Top the tortillas with 1/3 of the grated veggie cheese followed by 1/3 of the spring onions and 1/3 of the olives. Sprinkle with garlic and chili powder to taste.
4. Repeat layering the tortillas, veggie cheese, spring onions, olives and seasoning completing 2 more layers.
5. Bake in the oven for approximately 5 minutes or until the soya cheese has melted.
6. Remove from the oven and serve immediately with a side of your favorite salsa or guacamole.
7. Enjoy!

How To Make Pita Chips

You can use your favorite pita bread as an alternative to tortilla chips. Simply cut the pita bready in triangle shaped pieces, approximately the same size as a tortilla chip and toast them in a toaster oven until crispy.

Ingredients

1 large bag of organic blue corn tortillas (available at health store)

1 brick of grated veggie cheddar cheese

1/3 cup of finely chopped spring onions

1/3 cup of green or black olives depending you what you prefer

Garlic powder to taste –"Garlic Plus" is a good spice

Chili powder to taste

Amazing Tofu Curry

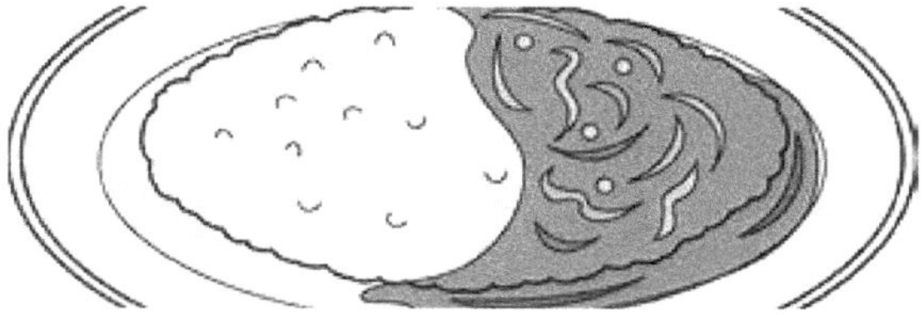

From: Mom-G

Prep Time: 2 days

Serves: 6

Cook Time: 20 min

Instructions

1. Dice tofu into large chunks (approx. 1") and season in salt, onion, garlic and black pepper for about 2 days.
2. Mix the nutmeg, cinnamon, cloves, salt, curry powder, cumin and paprika with enough water to make a paste and fry in a large pot in 2 tbsp of oil for a two minutes.
3. Add tofu and potatoes and let simmer in the paste on low heat for 10 minutes stirring constantly.
4. Add enough water to cover the tofu and ½ cup of coconut milk and cook on low heat for about an hour.
5. Serve on a bed of rice or quinoa with naan bread.
6. Enjoy!

Ingredients

1 pkg firm tofu

1 small onion diced

4 cloves garlic diced

½ tsp nutmeg

½ tsp cinnamon

½ tsp cloves

2 tsp curry powder

1 tbsp cumin

1 tsp paprika

1 tsp sea salt or Himalayan salt

2 potatoes diced (to thicken the sauce)

Black pepper to taste

Delicious Aromatic Curry

Curry powder is actually a mixture of a number of other spices. Generally, curry powder is a combination of cumin, turmeric, ground ginger, black pepper, ground coriander and chili powder (ground cardamom is sometimes used also).

Individually the spices in curry powder offer some health benefits. Combined they boast many benefits including boosting your metabolism, aiding in digestion, promoting good heart health and the turmeric in the curry powder can aid in pain and inflammation relief.

Garlic Tofu & Noodles

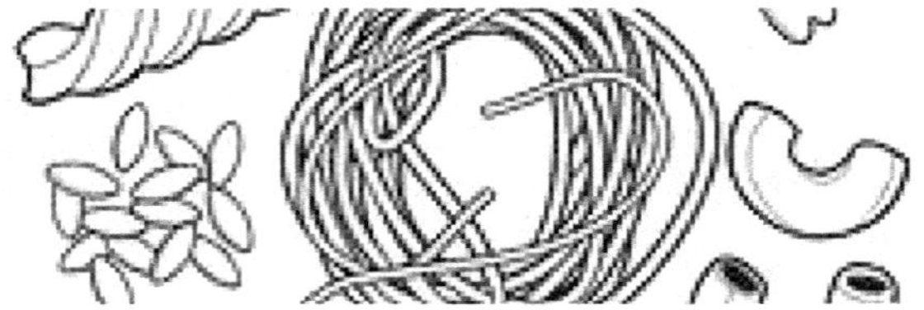

From: Mom-G

Serves: 4—6

Prep Time: 2 day marinate and 5 min

Cook Time: 20 min

Ingredients

1 pkg brown rice penne pasta or any pasta

1 tbsp soy sauce

1 tsp garlic powder

1 pkg extra firm tofu

handful small mushrooms

1 red bell pepper roasted

dried oregano to taste

salt to taste

fresh parsley – to your liking

1 medium onion diced

Instructions

1. Dice tofu and season with soy sauce, onion powder, garlic powder and black pepper (to taste) and let marinade for 2 days in the fridge prior to cooking.
2. Boil pasta to desired texture, strain and set aside.
3. Meanwhile, fry tofu until brown. Add mushrooms, bell peppers and onions and cook for about ten minutes.
4. Add pasta, oregano, garlic powder and parsley and toss while cooking for five minutes.

Press it out!

Pressing excess moisture out of your tofu makes it firmer and thirsty—better able to absorb the delicious marinade.

Poppy's Best Vegan Quiche

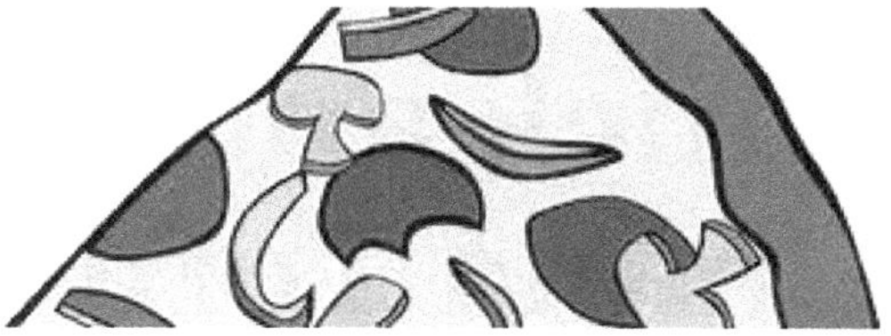

Serves: 4 to 6

Prep Time: 20 min

Cook Time: 50-60 min

Ingredients

1 medium onion chopped

6-8 mushrooms sliced (optional)

3 cloves of garlic

1 tbsp olive oil

8oz frozen prepared pastry (or make your own—see recipe for Perfect Pastry)

3/4 block firm tofu

2 tsp oat milk

1 tbsp lemon juice

1 tsp sea salt

1 tsp black pepper

1 tsp garlic powder

1 tsp onion powder

1 tsp paprika

1 cup shredded vegan cheese

3 tomatoes sliced

Instructions

1. Preheat the oven to 400 degrees.
2. Cook the onion, mushrooms and garlic in oil until tender (approx. 3-5 minutes).
3. Press the pastry into a 9" dish and bake 5 minutes.
4. Using your hands, crumble the tofu into a food processor, this will make it easier to bend. Blend the tofu using a food processor. Add oat milk , lemon juice and spices and continue to blend until a thick creamy texture is achieved.
5. Transfer the blended tofu mixture to a large bowl and incorporate the onions and garlic and vegan cheese and mix well.
6. Spoon into baked pastry.
7. Layer the sliced tomatoes across the top of the quiche.
8. Bake for 50 minutes until done. Cover the quiche with aluminum foil for the first 40 minutes of baking then remove.
9. Allow quiche to cool for 10—15 minutes before cutting.
10. Serve with a fresh, organic salad
11. Enjoy

More pressing matters...

Pressing excess moisture out of your tofu makes it firmer and thirsty—better able to absorb the delicious marinade.

Quick and Easy Chana Tofu Curry

Serves: 4

Prep Time: 45 min

Cook Time: 20 min

Instructions

1. In a large saucepan, fry onions and garlic until golden on medium high.
2. Add curry powder, fry for another minute.
3. Add in potatoes, chickpeas and tofu and cup of water, mix well. Reduce to low medium heat and cover. Cook for another 20 minutes. Add salt and pepper to taste.
4. Add more water for more sauce. Mash many potatoes for a thicker sauce.
5. Check to make sure potatoes are soft by pressing with a fork, if they are soft curry is ready.
6. Serve on bed of brown basmati rice with warm naan bread (like an airy pita bread) or papadums (crispy lentil bread).

Healing Spices

All ingredients in curry are fabulous healing herbs!

Prepared curry powders are available mild to hot, start with mild if you are unsure you can always add more curry or chili peppers.

Ingredients

2 tbsp prepared Curry Powder

1 can organic chick peas

1 package extra firm organic tofu

1 onion finely chopped

2-3 cloves of garlic finely sliced

2 large potatoes peeled and chopped 1" cubes

1 tsp sea salt

Organic black pepper

1 cup water

2 cups brown basmati rice (follow instructions on package)

Praise Seitan Steaks

Serves: 4

Worth the time :)

Prep Time: 4.5 hours

Cook Time: 20 min

Instructions

1. In a large mixing bowl, mash the kidney beans and black beans.
2. Add the soy sauce, tomato sauce, nutritional yeast and spices and mix well by hand.
3. Add vital wheat gluten and mix well until the mixture appears dry and crumbly.
4. Slowly drizzle in the vegetable broth over the mixture while stirring with a fork. Mix as thoroughly as possible with a fork until the mixture is firm but slightly sticky.
5. Use hands to knead the dough until all ingredients have been completely incorporated (about 4-5 minutes). The mixture should form in to a firm ball.
6. Divide the dough into four even pieces. Using a rolling pin roll each piece into steak like shapes approximately a 1/2 inch thick.
7. Using a steaming pan, steam the steaks for 50 minutes flipping them over at 25 minutes.
8. In the meantime, place all of the marinade ingredients in a blender and blend until smooth.
9. Once out of the steamer place the steaks in a large pan and coat thoroughly with the marinade, cover with plastic wrap and let sit in the fridge for at least 3 hours.
10. When the steaks have properly marinated, heat two tablespoons of olive oil in a fry pan and fry each steak over medium heat until golden brown.

FYI

You can cut the steaks up into small pieces and freeze them to be used later in stir fry's, burritos or other dishes— if they last that long....

Ingredients

1 tsp black pepper

1 tsp onion powder

1/4 canned black beans

1/4 canned kidney beans

2 tbsp soy sauce

2 1/2 tbsp tomato sauce

3 tbsp nutritional yeast

1 tsp smoked paprika

2 tsp garlic powder

1/2 tsp ground rosemary

1/2 tsp fine sea salt

1/2 cup vegetable broth

1 1/2 cup vital wheat gluten

Marinade

3 tbsp of soy sauce

3 tbsp of Dijon mustard

4 cloves of garlic

1 tsp of smoked paprika

1 tsp black pepper

1 tbsp of barbeque sauce

Traditional Dhal

From: Mom-G

Serves: 2 to 3

Prep Time: 25 min

Cook Time: 20 min

Ingredients

4 cups water

1 cup split peas

1 tsp turmeric

1 onion diced

4 cloves garlic diced

Salt to taste

1 tbsp cumin roasted

½ red bell pepper roasted

Instructions

1. Bring water to a boil. Add split peas, salt and all of the ingredients.
2. Cook until split peas are mushy.
3. Add roasted cumin once the peas are mushy and cook for a few more minutes.
4. Serve hot.

Roasted Cumin

Cumin can be roasted in small fry pan on low heat with no oil. Roast on pan for about 1 minute until fragrant. Do not let burn.

Side & Veggie

Side Dish *noun*— **A dish that is served with but subordinate to Entrée or Main course**

1: Simple Stuffed Red Peppers

2: Tomato Basil Side

3: Sautéed Kale

4: Grilled Asparagus Tips

5: Broccoli Cauliflower Side

6: Enoki Mushroom Tempura

7: Smashed Sweet Potatoes

8: Brown Basmati Rice and Pine Nut Stuffing

9: Roasted Portobello Mushrooms

Simple Stuffed Red Peppers

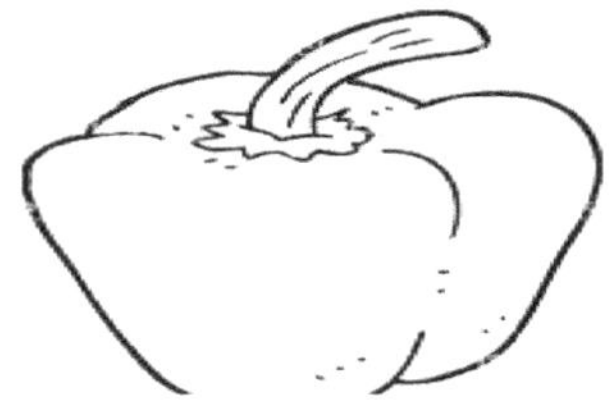

Serves: 4

Prep Time: 15 min

Cook Time: 15—20 min

Instructions

1. Cut top off the red peppers and remove the seeds and white inners.
2. Cook brown rice according to instructions on package along with peas tomato paste and bouillon.
3. Mix in coriander leaves and nutritional yeast.
4. Stuff mixture into the peppers. Sprinkle a little nutritional yeast on top of peppers.
5. Place in low baking dish. Bake stuffed peppers at 350F for 15 – 20 minutes.
6. Serve with fresh mixed salad.
7. Enjoy

Pick a Pepper

There are over 50, 000 estimated types of peppers. Of these one of the most common are Bell peppers. An unknown fact to many is that green peppers are unmatured or unripe red peppers.

Therefore, green peppers only contain about half the vitamin C and a fraction of the vitamin A contained in an orange or red pepper.

Green peppers also tend to be more bitter because they have not had a chance to properly ripen.

Bell peppers promote eye health and can aid in increasing your metabolic rate.

Ingredients

4 red peppers

1 cup brown rice

1 cup shelled green peas or edamame

2 tbsp tomato paste

2 tbsp chopped coriander leaves (can substitute with parsley)

1 tsp chili powder

4 tbsp Nutritional yeast

1 bouillon cube

Tomato Basil Side

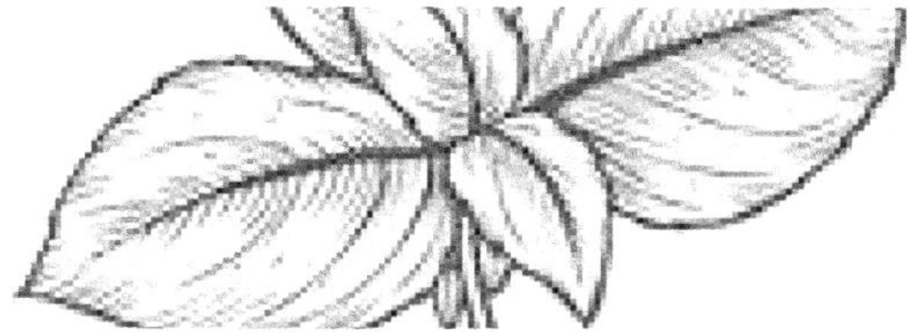

Serves: 2 to 4 Prep Time: 10 min

Ingredients

4 firm large room temperature tomatoes

1/2 cup fresh basil leaves chopped

2 tbsp olive oil

1/2 tsp sea salt

black pepper to taste

2 tbsp pesto sauce or to taste

Instructions

1. Wash and core tomatoes. Slice width-wise 1/4 ".
2. Display across platter with overlap.
2. Spread pesto down centre of sliced tomatoes.
3. Sprinkle basil leaves on top, add salt and pepper.
4. Drizzle olive oil all over.
5. Serve and enjoy!

Basilico

This flavor packed herb can be used to add a unique taste to any dish. Typically used in pesto, pasta and other Mediterranean dishes, this plant is believed to originate in Southeast Asia.

High in zinc, iron, calcium and vitamins A and C , this healthy plant help lower blood sugar and cholesterol.

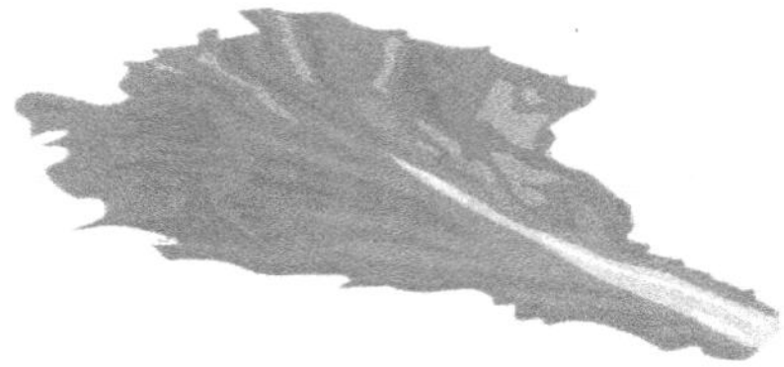

Sauteed Kale

Serves: 4

Prep Time: 10 min

Cook Time: 2-5 min

Ingredients

1 bunch of kale, rinsed and coarsely chopped

2 tbsp extra virgin olive oil

1/2 large organic lemon

3 cloves of organic garlic, thinly sliced

Sea salt to taste

Ground organic black pepper to taste

Instructions

1. In a large sauté pan heat olive oil over medium high heat.
2. Add the garlic and sauté until tender, approximately two minutes.
3. Add kale, sauté another three minutes until wilted and bright green.
4. Add lemon, sea salt and ground pepper to taste, toss gently, serve and enjoy!

Kale ya!

Available in a number of varieties, Kale which is a member of the cabbage family is densely packed with vitamins and minerals such as Vitamins A, B6, C, K , calcium, magnesium and potassium to name just a few.

Grilled Asparagus Tips

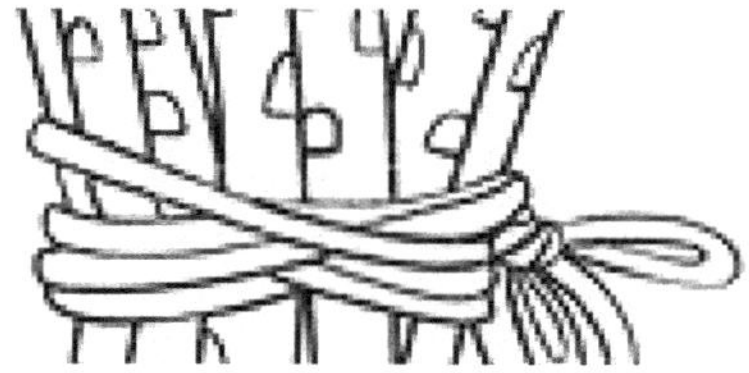

Serves: 4 to 6

Prep Time: 10 min

Cook Time: 6– 8 min

Ingredients

2 lb asparagus, stalks trimmed

2 tbsp olive oil

1 lemon—juice squeezed

1 tsp sea salt or Himalayan salt

1/2 tsp black pepper

2 tbsp Vegasan—optional (see Sauces & Dressings)

Instructions

1. On a baking sheet, spread out asparagus.
2. Sprinkle salt and pepper over all.
3. Drizzle olive oil over all and fresh lemon juice.
4. Roll asparagus with hands to make sure all are covered with oil.
5. Place asparagus on grill. Turn after 3 minutes, grill another 3 minutes. Take off grill when tips turning brown.
6. Add Vegasan for cheezy flavour (optional).
7. Serve immediately.
8. Enjoy!

FYI

The best way to trim asparagus stalks is to hold in both hands and let it snap where it wants. This will leave you with the tender, delicious part of the asparagus.

Asparagus

Asparagus belongs to the Liliaceae family of foods. Other vegetables in this family include leeks, onions, chives and garlic. Low in calories, asparagus is a fiber rich food containing brain nourishing folic acid, potassium and vitamin A.

Broccoli Cauliflower Side

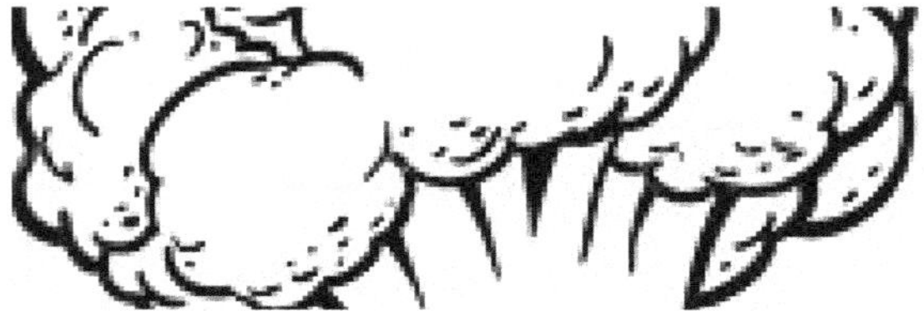

Serves: 6 Prep Time: 20 min

Ingredients

2 cups broccoli small pieces

2 cups cauliflower small pieces

1/2 cup chopped celery

1/4 chopped red onion

1 cup of fresh or frozen green peas

1/4 cup shredded carrots

1 1/4 Vegan-Naise (see Sauces & Dressings)

1/8 tsp salt

1 tbsp sugar

1 tsp vinegar

paprika to taste

Instructions

1. Mix together broccoli, cauliflower, celery, onion, peas and carrots in large bowl.
2. Mix together Vegan-Naise, sugar, salt and vinegar in separate bowl.
3. Add to vegetable mixture and toss well. Allow to marinate together for one hour.
4. Sprinkle paprika on top. Enjoy!

FYI

This is a great side but could also be made as a meal :)

Enoki Mushroom Tempura

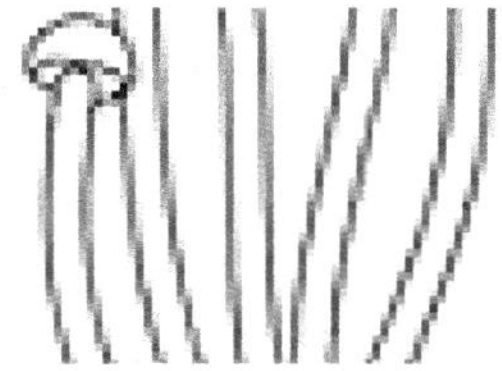

Serves: 2 to 3

Prep Time: 20 min

Cook Time: 20 min

Ingredients

1 cup of all purpose flour

1 egg replacer (ground flax works too, 1 tsp to 2 tbsp water and let sit)

1 cup of ice water (4 ice cubes to cool the water)

1 tsp smoked paprika

1 tsp garlic powder

1 tsp onion powder

3 cups of vegetable oil for frying

1 pack of Enoki mushrooms

Instructions

1. In a large bowl prepare your egg replacer.
2. Add the iced water making sure not to add the ice cubes and mix thoroughly.
3. In a separate bowl combine the flour and spices.
4. Add the flour and spice mixture to the water and egg replacer mixture slowly. Combine using a whisk being careful not to over mix. The mixture should be slightly lumpy.
5. In a medium sized wok or pot heat up the vegetable oil to about 180°.
6. While the oil is heating up, wash and dry the Enoki mushrooms. Using a knife remove most of the root, leaving enough to hold the mushrooms clumped together. Separate the mushrooms into bite sized clumps.
7. Using chopsticks, dip each bite sized portion of mushrooms into the tempura batter then place in hot oil. You can fry a few portions at a time but not too many so they do not stick together. Fry the mushrooms until golden brown and remove from oil
8. Place on a plate lined with a paper towel to absorb excess oil. Once all of the mushrooms have been fried, lightly salt. You can serve the mushrooms with your favorite

Enoki, Enoki! Who's there?

These delicately flavored mild mushrooms are perfect for frying. Enoki mushrooms grow in clusters from a single root. They have long stems with a small cap.

Smashed Sweet Potatoes

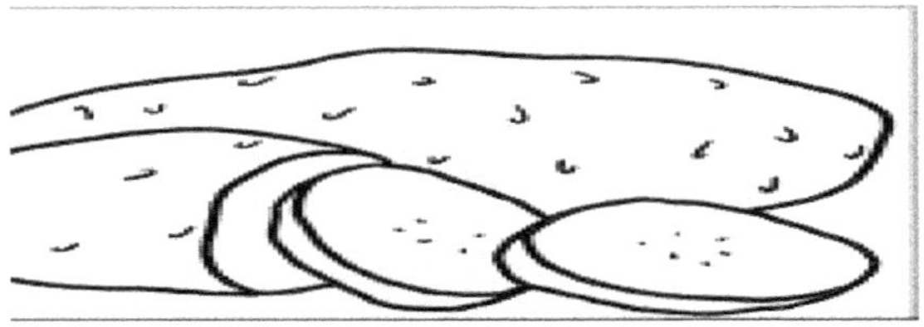

Serves: 4 to 6

Prep Time: 15 min

Cook Time: 45 min

Ingredients

5 sweet potatoes

1 tbsp miso paste

2 tsp maple syrup

1 tsp ground cinnamon

Instructions

1. Preheat oven to 350 F. Bake the sweet potatoes for 45 minutes or until tender.
2. Cool, peel, skin and transfer to large bowl.
3. Mash with potato masher, add miso, maple syrup and cinnamon. Mash until desired consistency.
4. Enjoy!

Sweet Sweet Potato

These sweet tasting root vegetables are a healthier option to potatoes. Contrary to the effects of potatoes on the diet, sweet potatoes can aid in weight loss. High in Vitamin A, they are beneficial to your skin, bones and help to improve vision. They also support the immune system.

Brown Basmati Rice and Pine Nut Stuffing

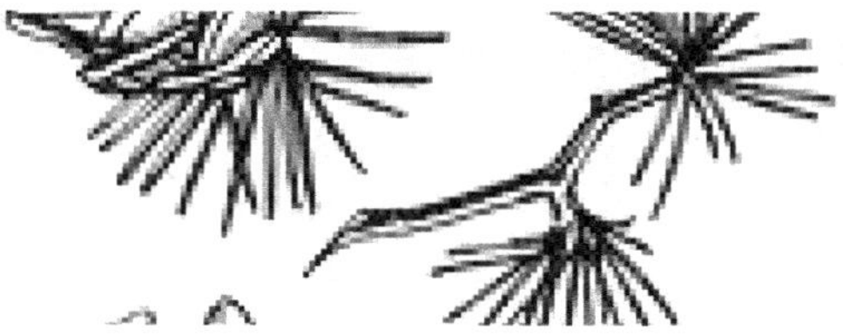

Serves: 4 to 6

Prep Time: 15 min

Cook Time: 20 min

Ingredients

1 cup brown basmati rice

2 organic vegetable broth cubes

1 cup pine nuts

1/2 large onion, chopped

2 tbsp soy bacon bits

1/2 tsp ground black pepper

2 tbsp Olive oil

Instructions

1. Cook basmati rice according to instructions and add vegetable cubes to boiling water.
2. Fry onions on medium high heat until brown in olive oil for approximately 5 minutes add soy bits for the last minute.
3. In separate pan, roast pine nuts on medium heat (no oil added), until brown.
4. Mix cooked rice, onion, soy bits, and roasted pine nuts together.
5. Add black pepper.
6. Enjoy!

Roasted Portobello Mushrooms

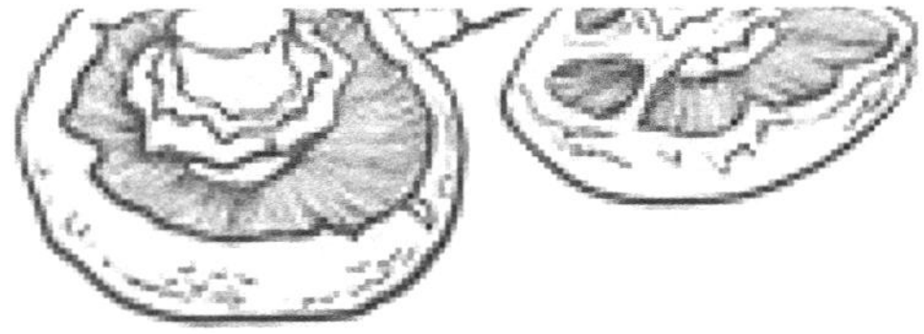

Serves: 4 to 8

Prep Time: 10min

Cook Time: 10 min

Ingredients

4 large portobello mushrooms

4 tsp tamari sauce

6 tsp Organic Olive oil

8 drops Liquid Smoke

Instructions

1. Wash mushrooms and gently remove stems, discard stems.
2. Rub olive oil mixed with liquid smoke gently over top and bottom of mushrooms.
3. Place mushrooms on baking sheet gill sides up. Drizzle remaining olive oil and tamari on top.
4. Bake for 10 minutes at 400F in oven until tender.
5. Enjoy!

Sauces & Dressings

Sauces *noun*—Flavourful relish or dressing or topping that is served as an accompaniment to food

Herbed Vinaigrette

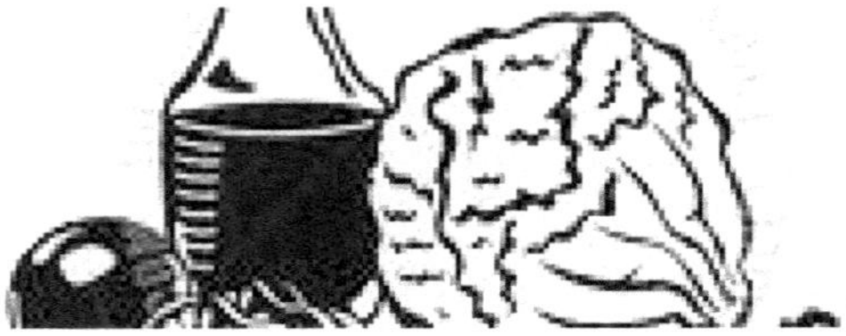

Serves: 6+ Prep Time: 15 min

Ingredients

2 cups of extra-virgin olive oil

1 cup of white wine vinegar

1 tablespoon Dijon mustard

1 tablespoon of dried thyme

1 tablespoon of dried tarragon

1 tablespoon of dried oregano

1 ½ teaspoon of sea salt

1 teaspoon of freshly ground black pepper

¼ cup fresh lemon juice

¼ cup chopped parsley

Instructions

1. Put all of the ingredients in a blender.
2. Blend until well combined.

Tarragon & Oregano

Tarragon, believed to originate in Siberia, is a beautiful , aromatic herb used to add zest to most foods. The health benefits of this herb includes, aiding in digestion, supporting heart health, aiding in regulating blood sugar and tarragon is a natural diuretic.

Surprisingly, the oregano plant belongs to the mint family despite their contrasting tastes. The health benefits of this herb have been gaining popularity over the last decade with properties making it anti-inflammatory, anti-bacterial, anti-viral and oregano is high in antioxidants.

Mia Italian Dressing

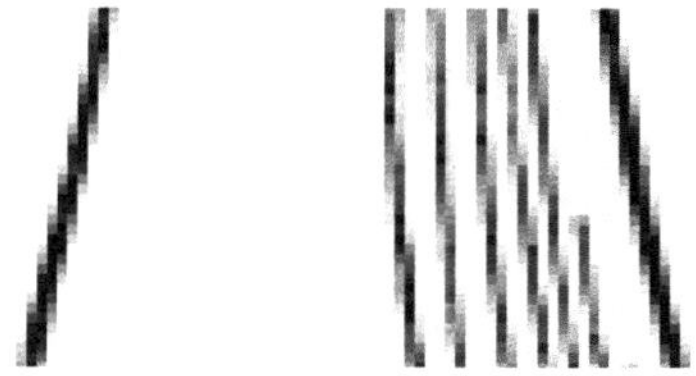

Serves: 4+ Prep Time: 5 min

Ingredients

2 cloves garlic, minced

1 tsp dried tarragon

1 tsp dried marjoram

1 tsp dry mustard

1/2 tsp sea salt

1/4 tsp pepper

1/2 cup olive oil

2 tbsp red wine vinegar

Instructions

1. Combine all the ingredients in a jar with a tight lid.
2. Shake the jar well and let stand for one hour at room temperature, chill.
3. Shake well before serving.

Mustard in History

This culinary staple has a long history but it was not in the kitchen. Historically mustard was used for medicinal purposes. It was widely used topically to heal sores, and congestions in the form of mustard packs.

While there are more than 40 varieties of mustard plants, there are 5 main types of mustard widely used for cooking.

Experiment with all of them to see which ones suit your taste buds.

Tahini Lemon Dressing

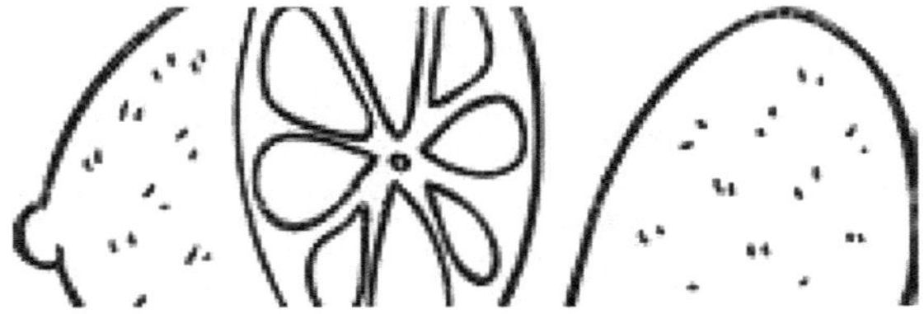

Serves: 3+ Prep Time: 10 min

Ingredients

1/2 cup lemon juice

1/2 cup olive oil

1/3 cup tahini

2 tbsp agave

2 cloves garlic, minced

1 tsp sea salt

1/2 tsp ground pepper

Instructions

1. Combine lemon juice, olive oil, tahini, agave, and garlic in blender. Blend until smooth.
2. Season with salt and pepper.
3. Enjoy!

Vegan-Naise

Serves: many Prep Time: 15 min

Ingredients

1 cup sunflower or safflower oil

1/2 cup soy milk (room temperature)

1tsp Dijon mustard

2 tsp lemon juice

1/4 tsp sea salt

Instructions

1. Put all ingredients in a medium bowl. Blend with an emersion blender until it becomes creamy, approximately 20 seconds.
2. Add more oil if it does not thicken.
3. Keep in a sealed jar, it will last for a week in the refrigerator.
4. Enjoy!

Multi-use Vegan-Naise

Can be used as a spread or base for dips. For dips add garlic, hot sauces or any of your preferred sauces.

Vegasan

Serves: many

Prep Time: 10 min

Ingredients

1/2 cup nutritional yeast

1/2 cup finally ground almonds

1/2 tsp sea salt

1/2 tsp onion powder

1/4 tsp garlic powder

Instructions

1. In a medium sized jar, add all ingredients.
2. Shake all ingredients together with lid on.
3. Presto! Instant Vegasan!
4. Serve on anything where you want a "cheezy" flavour!
5. Will last a long time in the fridge!

Shake it up, shake it on!

This is your vegan parmesan. It is great on pasta, popcorn, veggies, and more!

Fiery Chipotle Dip

Serves: many

Prep Time: 10min

Refrigeration: 1 hour

Instructions

1. Place all ingredients into blender and mix until the texture is smooth and refrigerate approximately an hour to thicken.
2. This dip goes with tortilla chips, veggies, crackers, and more. Also can be used as a spread or salad dressing.
3. This dip will keep in the refrigerator for a week
4. Enjoy!

Ingredients

1 block silken tofu

1/2 cup safflower oil

juice of half lemon

3 tbsp agave nectar or maple syrup

2 tbsp apple cider vinegar

1/2 cup red onions

1 tsp sea salt

3 cloves of garlic minced

2 tbsp nutritional yeast

1/2 tsp chili powder

1 tbsp drained capers

2 chipotle peppers (less if you don't want too much spice or more if you like it hot)

Dulcé

Dulce verb—To make sweet to soothe.

Brown Rice Pudding

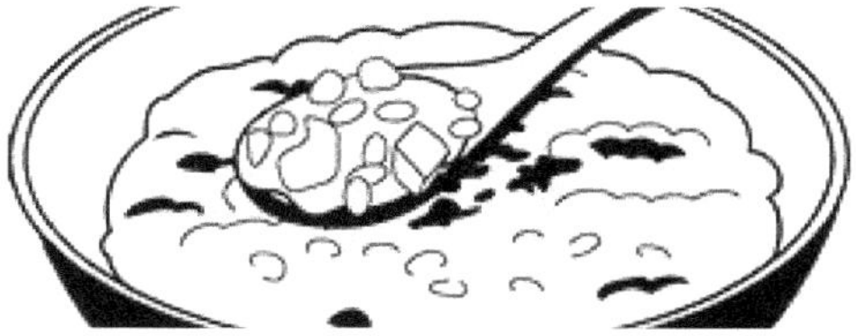

Serves: 4

Prep Time: 1hr

Cook Time: 1hr

Ingredients

1 ½ cups of brown rice

½ teaspoon of sea salt (fine grained)

2 tablespoons of arrowroot powder

(or corn starch)

1 tablespoon of ground cinnamon

1 ½ cups of oat milk or any nut milk

¼ cup maple syrup

¼ cup raisins (optional)

Instructions

1. Preheat the oven to 350 F.
2. Bring the brown rice and 3 cups of water to a boil in a medium saucepan. Once it is boiling reduce heat to low, cover and simmer for 40 – 50 minutes, or until the rice is very soft.
3. In a large bowl, dissolve the arrowroot powder (or corn starch) in 1 cup of the oat milk. Then add the rice, raisins, maple syrup, cinnamon, and salt and mix well.
4. Pour the mixture into a large greased baking dish, cover with foil and bake for 1 hour, or until lightly brown and bubbly.
5. Remove from the oven and stir in the remaining ½ cup of oat milk. Leave the pudding to cool for about 1 hour before serving.
6. Add your favorite toppings and enjoy!

Note:

This is a delicious yet healthy dish that can be served for breakfast or as a late evening desert. It can be topped with any one of your favorite toppings such as cinnamon, blueberries, maple syrup, toasted nuts or anything else you like.

Cinnamon & Maple Syrup R Good 4 U

Cinnamon is great for enhancing any recipe but this tasty sweet spice is also important for its many health benefits. Cinnamon can help to lower cholesterol and lower blood sugar levels. Cinnamon has also been proven to reduce inflammation.

When you think of maple syrup you probably think of it being high in sugar and calories, but did you know that maple syrup is also a good a good source of manganese and zinc, it is also an antioxidant and known to boost the immune system.

Christmas Cookies

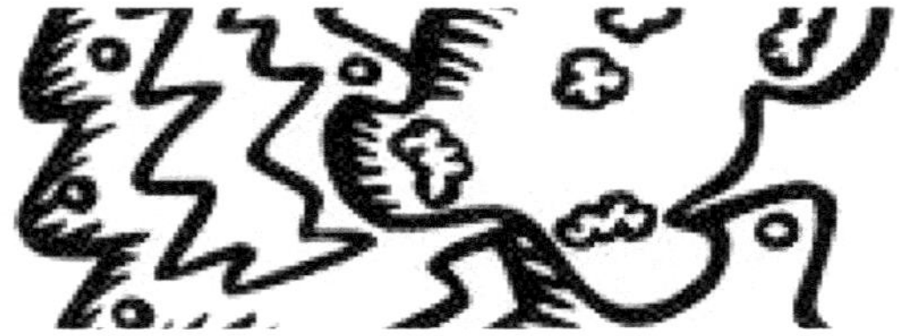

Serves: Many

Prep Time: 3hrs,25 min

Cook Time: 6 min

Instructions

1. In a large bowl, mix the vegan margarine and sugar until creamy. Mix in the egg replacer, molasses, and vinegar. Set aside.
2. In a medium bowl, sift together the dry ingredients. Add to the wet ingredients.
3. Chill in the refrigerator for 3 hours or overnight.
4. Preheat the oven to 375°F. Lightly grease a cookie sheet.
5. Remove from the refrigerator and roll out on a floured surface. Cut into desired shapes (stars, trees, stockings, etc.).
6. Bake for 6 to 8 minutes, until the edges brown. Cool for 5 minutes on the cookie sheet and remove to a wire rack.
7. While the cookies are cooling, make the frosting. Using a hand mixer, cream the vegan margarine. Add the shortening and continue to mix. Add the remaining ingredients and mix until thoroughly combined. The frosting should be stiff.
8. Using a pastry bag and a star tip, decorate the cookies.

Makes about 3 dozen yummy cookies. Enjoy!!

Egg Replacers

Egg replacers/egg substitutes are the perfect replacement for eggs in any recipe and can be found in most health food and grocery stores. *Special note – one teaspoon of ground flaxseed and one tablespoon of water can be used as a substitute for one egg.

Ingredients

Cookies

1 cup vegan margarine
1 cup sugar
egg replacer (equivalent to 1 egg)
1 cup molasses
2 tbsp organic apple cider vinegar
5 cups flour
½ tsp salt
1 ½ tsp baking soda
1 tbsp ginger
1 ¼ tsp cinnamon
1 tsp ground cloves

Frosting

½ cup vegan margarine
½ cup vegetable shortening
4 cups powdered sugar
1 ½ tsp vanilla
1 tbsp vanilla plant milk
food coloring of your choice

Dulcé

Delicious Jeezcake

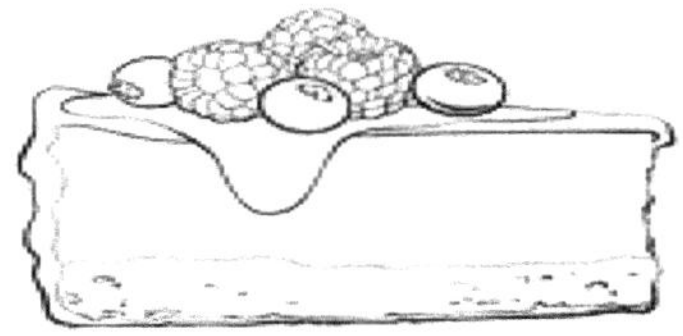

Serves: 4-8

Prep Time: 15 min

Cook Time: 25-35 min

Ingredients

The Crust

2 tbsp vegetable margarine

1 tbsp water

1 ¾ cups of organic granola

The Filling

2 lbs soft tofu

2 ½ tbsp of lemon juice

¾ of maple syrup or granulated sugar

1/3 cup of sunflower oil

1 tbsp of vanilla extract

2 tsp of lemon zest

1 cup of chocolate chips

Instructions

1. Blend the granola in a food processor breaking it up in to a powder.
2. Melt the margarine and add to the food processor along with the water and blend until well mixed. If the texture is still very crumbly, add an additional tablespoon of water.
3. Press the mixture firmly into an 8 or 10 inch pie pan, and bake for approximately 8 to 10 minutes.
4. Blend all of the ingredients except the chocolate chips in a blender or food processor and process until smooth.
5. Fold the chocolate chips into the mixture then pour all of the filling into the crust and bake for 25 to 35 minutes. The top of the cheesecake should spring back at a light touch.
6. Cool the cheesecake completely before slicing. As the cheesecake cools it will become firmer.
7. Serve this cheesecake as is or topped with your favorite fruit and enjoy!

Delicious Substitute

This recipe is sure to be a favorite not only for those who may be lactose intolerant, but anyone looking for a delicious and easy to make desert.

Quick & Cheezy Cookies

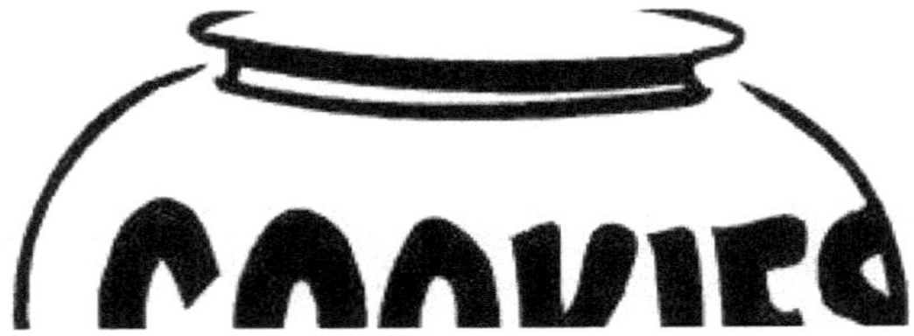

Serves: 4+

Prep Time: 35 min

Cook Time: 10 min

Instructions

1. Mix all ingredients and chill for approximately ½ hour
2. Shape into a roll and slice ¼".
3. Place on cookie sheet and bake for 10 minutes at 400F.
4. Enjoy!

Ingredients

1 cup all purpose flour

½ tsp paprika

¼ tsp dry mustard

cayenne powder to taste

½ cup vegetable margarine

2 cup shredded vegan cheese

Dulcé

Peanut Butter & Chocolate Marble Fudge

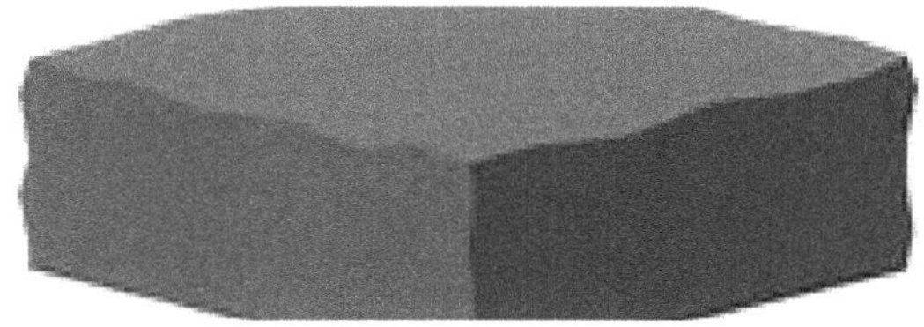

Serves: 4+

Prep Time: 25 min

Chill Time: 3 hr

Ingredients

Peanut Butter Fudge

½ cup of organic peanut butter

½ cup cashews

¼ cup agave nectar

3 tablespoons of coconut oil

½ a teaspoon of vanilla extract

Chocolate Fudge

1/4 cup of cocoa powder

1 cup cashews

¼ cup agave nectar

3 tablespoons of coconut oil

½ a teaspoon of vanilla extract

½ teaspoon of salt

Instructions

1. Chocolate Fudge: Blend cashews in a food processor until buttery with no lumps. Add cocoa and salt and continue to blend. Add agave nectar, coconut oil, and vanilla and blend until thoroughly combined, at this point it should begin to ball up. Remove from the processor and set aside.
2. Peanut Butter Fudge: Blend cashews in a food processor as before until you reach the desired texture. Add cocoa and salt and continue to blend. Add peanut butter, agave nectar, coconut oil, and vanilla and blend until thoroughly combined.
3. Cut each ball of dough into 4 large chunks so you have 8 in total. Begin to marble fudge by combining one chuck of chocolate fudge with one chunk of peanut butter fudge together, and knead until you see it marbling. Continue adding another chunk alternating between chocolate fudge and peanut butter fudge until you have used up all 8 pieces.
4. Press the marbled fudge into a one inch thick flat rectangle in a Pyrex dish. Chill covered in fridge overnight or for at least 3 hours.
5. Enjoy!

FYI. This is delicious dairy free fudge is very easy to make, tastes awesome and you won't feel guilty about having a second, third or fourth piece!

PB & Cashews

More than just being delicious, peanut butter is a good source of fiber, potassium, healthy fats. Not to mention that it is very high in protein.

You probably already know that cashews are high in protein but did you also know that they are good for heart health, may help to prevent gall stones, are a great antioxidant and a good source of magnesium making them a perfect nighttime snack.

Perfect Pumpkin Pie

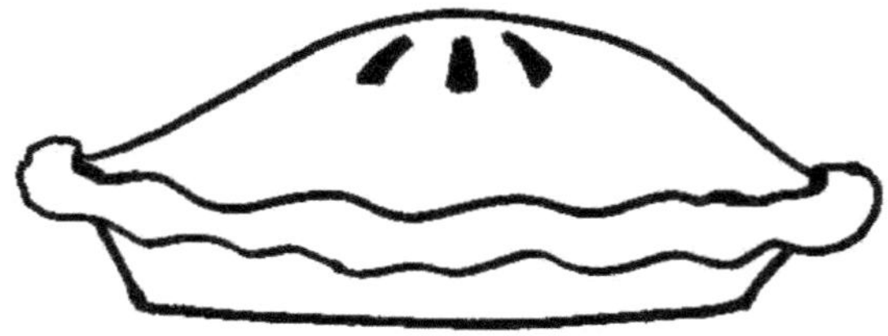

Serves: 4-8

Prep Time: 25 min

Cook Time: 1 hr

Ingredients

3/4 lb silken tofu
1 16-oz can pure pumpkin
1 1/2 tsp cinnamon
3/4 tsp ginger
1/2 tsp nutmeg
1 tsp salt
1/3 cup oil
1 tsp. vanilla
1 cup light brown sugar
1 1/2 tbsp molasses
1 unbaked 9-inch pastry crust (see Always Perfect Pastry to make your own)

Instructions

1. Preheat oven to 350°F.
2. Blend all ingredients except the pastry crust in a blender until smooth and creamy.
3. Pour this mixture into the unbaked pastry shell. (See recipe for always perfect pastry)
4. Bake for 1 hour.
5. Chill and serve.
6. Enjoy!!

Pumpkin & Molasses

Pumpkin is jammed with many health benefits including heart health, vision health, skin health, energy recovery after a workout and is also known to be an immune booster.

Here are some benefits of molasses you probably did not know. Molasses is known to be beneficial for constipation, arthritis, chronic fatigue syndrome, tumors and fibroids and anemia. Molasses is also an energy-booster.

The Super Hero Cookie

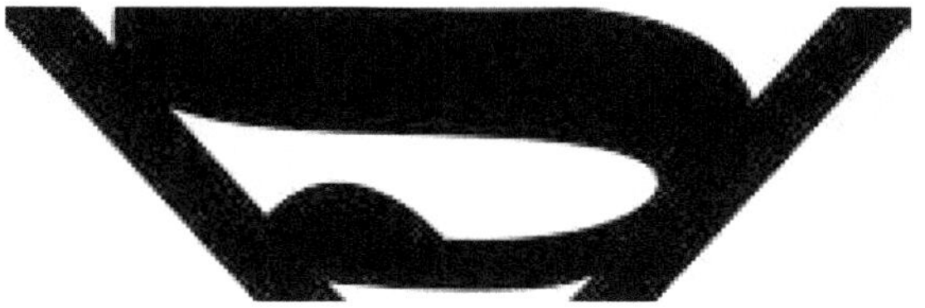

Serves: 4+

Prep Time: 45 min

Cook Time: 8-10 min

Instructions

1. Mix chia and water in a bowl and let sit for ½ hour.
2. Put **super mix 1** and **super mix 2** in food processor until well mixed.
3. Add all contents from the food processor into **super mix 3** and mix all together by hand.
4. Place a tablespoon of dough an inch apart on a coconut oiled cookie sheet pan.
5. Preheat oven 375 F and bake for 8 – 10 minutes.
6. Enjoy this healthy, delicious, energy-packed super cookie any time of the day!!

Ingredients

Super Mix #1

2 tbsp chia seed

6 tbsp spring water

Super Mix #2

1/2 cup organic coconut oil

1 cup coconut sugar

2 tsp vanilla extract

1 tsp baking soda

1/2 tsp ground cinnamon

1/4 tsp Himalayan salt

Super Mix #3

1 cup oat flour

2 cups quick flake oats

3/4 goji berries

1/4 raw cocoa beans

1 tbsp maca powder

Refreshing Fruit Salad

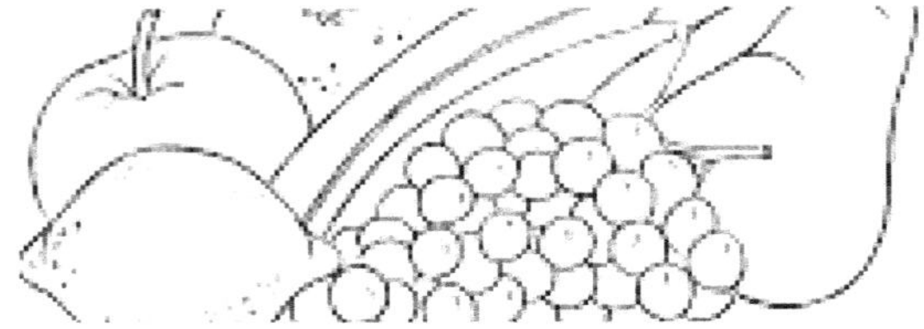

Serves: 4 Prep Time: 25 min

Ingredients

4 bananas sliced

1 cup of raspberry

1 cup of blueberry

1 cup sliced strawberries

2 cup chopped watermelon

2 cup chopped cantaloupe

2 red apples

1 pear

1 block silken tofu

2 tbsp agave nectar

1 pinch salt

1 tsp vanilla extract

½ cup slivered almonds, toasted lightly

Instructions

1. Put tofu in the blender add agave, vanilla extract, and a pinch of salt. Blend until smooth, then taste.
2. Adjust the sweetener, vanilla and salt to taste.
3. Mix all fruit in bowl and dish out onto individual plates. Put a couple spoonful's of the creamy tofu dressing on top and sprinkle the slivered almonds on the dressing.
4. Easy, delicious and nutritious! Enjoy!

Dulcé

Nana's Famous Chocolate Chip Cookies

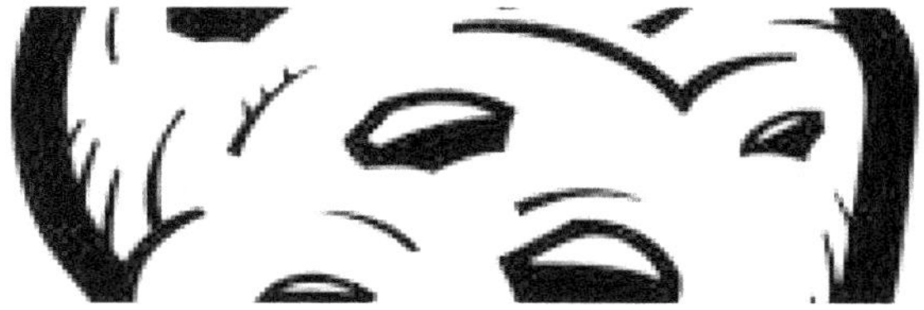

From: mommy

Prep Time: 25 min

Serves: many

Cook Time: 10 min

Ingredients

3/4 cup vegetable margarine

1 1/4 cup brown sugar

2 tbsp almond milk (or other nut milk)

1 tsp vanilla extract

1 tbsp white vinegar

1 tsp baking soda

1 3/4 cup flour

1 tsp salt

3/4 tsp baking soda

1 cup dark vegan chocolate chips

Instructions

1. Cream together vegetable margarine, brown sugar, almond milk and vanilla at medium speed with mixer.
2. Add in vinegar and baking soda, beat into mixture.
3. In a separate bowl, mix together flour, salt and second baking soda. Then slowly add to cream mixture at a low speed.
4. Stir in chocolate chips.
5. Roll into balls and place 2" apart on cookie sheet.

FYI

If you want a soft chewy cookie bake for 8 minutes, bake for 10 minutes if you want a crispy cookie.

Cookie dough can be made ahead of time and frozen. Take out when visitors come over.

Always Perfect Pastry

From: mommy
Prep Time: 25 min
Serves: many

Ingredients

5 cups of all purpose flour

2 tsp salt

1 lb vegetable shortening

1 1/2 tbsp vegetable oil, safflower is good

1 1/2 tbsp cold water

1 tsp baking powder

1 1/2 tbsp white vinegar

Instructions

1. Mix flour and salt together in large bowl.

2. Mix the shortening in with fingertips, rubbing in the flour until mealy.

3. In a separate bowl, mix oil, water, baking powder, and vinegar. Add more cold water to make 1 cup of liquid.

4. Mix both mixtures together. Chill mixture for about 20 minutes if too sticky to roll out.

Notes

Can be made into four balls and wrapped and frozen. Mixture will last for up to five days in the refrigerator.

Peanut Butter Chocolate Cheezecake Pie

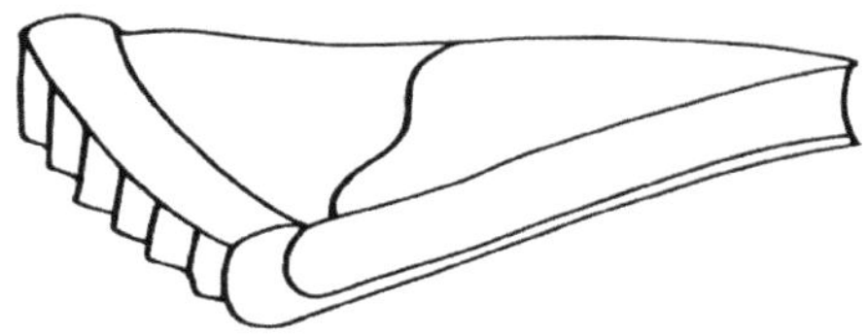

Prep Time: 3 hours

Serves: many

Instructions

1. Combine baking crumbs and melted margarine and press into a 9 inch pie pan. Cool in the refrigerator for 15 minutes.
2. In a large mixing bowl using a hand blender beat cream cheese, peanut butter and sugar until well combined.
3. Using a spatula fold in 1 cup of chocolate chips. Spoon the peanut butter, cream cheese mixture into the pie crust. Freeze for 1 hour before proceeding with the next step.
4. In a double broiler heat 1 cup of non-dairy chocolate chips until completely melted. Keeping the chocolate on low heat slowly drizzle the non-dairy milk in while whisking quickly and continuously to incorporate. Continue whisking until a thick creamy ganache is achieved.
5. Pour the warm ganache over the frozen pie and spread evenly over the top. Place in the refrigerator for at least one hour before serving.

Ingredients

Pie Crust

1 1/4 cups of Oreo baking crumbs.

(crumbs can be made by pulsing Oreo cookies in a blender— yes Oreos are vegan)

1/4 cup vegetable margarine

Pie Filling

2 packs of 227g non dairy cream cheese

1 cup of creamy peanut butter

1 cup granulated sugar

1 cups non-dairy chocolate chips

Ganache Topping

1 cups non-dairy chocolate chips

3/4 cups of any non dairy milk (more if required to achieve a creamy consistency)

Snacks & Nosh

Snack/nosh *noun*— A light, informal meal

1: Raw Energy Truffles

2: Raw Healthy Chocolate Bar

3: The Super Hero Cookie

4: Roasted Pumpkin Seeds

5: Kale Chips

6: Good Old Popped Corn

7: Perfect Pretzel

Raw Energy Truffles

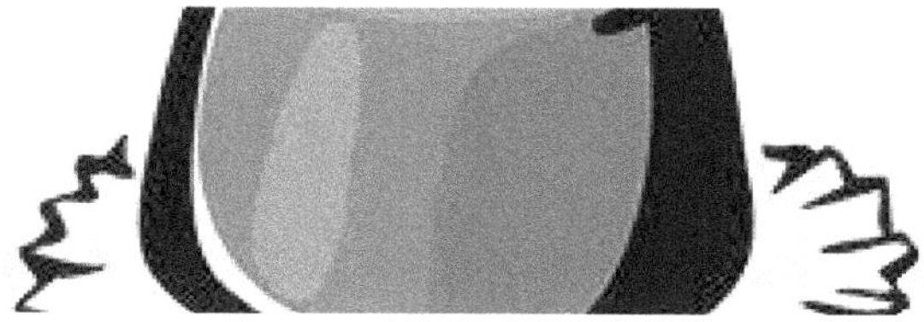

Serves: 2 to 3

Prep Time: 5-10 min

Ingredients

¼ cup raw cacao powder

1 cup organic walnuts

¼ cup maca powder

1 cup pitted dates

Pinch of sea salt or Himalayan salt

Pinch of cinnamon

Instructions

1. Blend all ingredients in a food processor until smooth.
2. Roll into balls.
3. For presentation, roll balls into shredded coconut or cocoa nibs or chopped nuts.

This is a quick, energy packed, nutritious treat! Enjoy!

The Wonderful Cocoa Bean

Full of antioxidants, the cocoa bean has many health benefits including improving heart health and brain function, lowers blood pressure, improves mood and increase insulin sensitivity which supports weight loss.

Raw Healthy Chocolate Bar

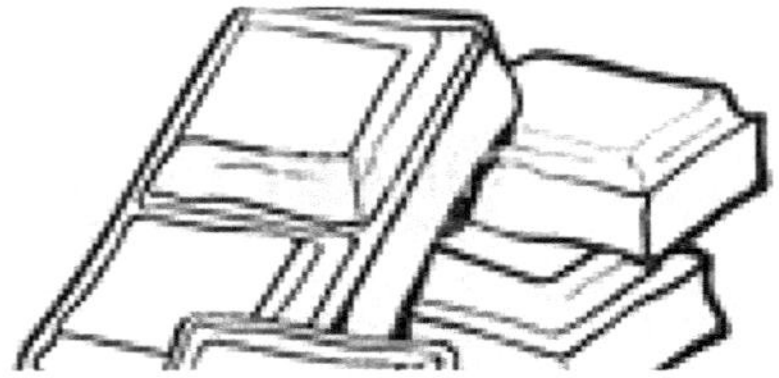

Serves: 1+

Prep Time: 10 min

Chill Time: 1 hr

Ingredients

1 tbsp virgin coconut oil

1 tbsp raw cacao powder

1 tsp raw almond butter

½ tsp maca root powder

½ tsp stevia

1 tbsp goji berries

1 tbsp or cocoa nibs

Instructions

1. Heat up a medium sized bowl in hot water. Empty water and melt coconut oil in bowl.
2. Add all other ingredients, blend well with spoon and smooth in bottom of bowl.
3. Freeze for 1 hour.
4. Remove from freezer and break up with spoon to bit size pieces.

Guilt-Free and Delish!

This easy, guilt-free recipe is not only full of antioxidants, but will give you extreme energy and is excellent tasting! Enjoy!

Roasted Pumpkin Seeds

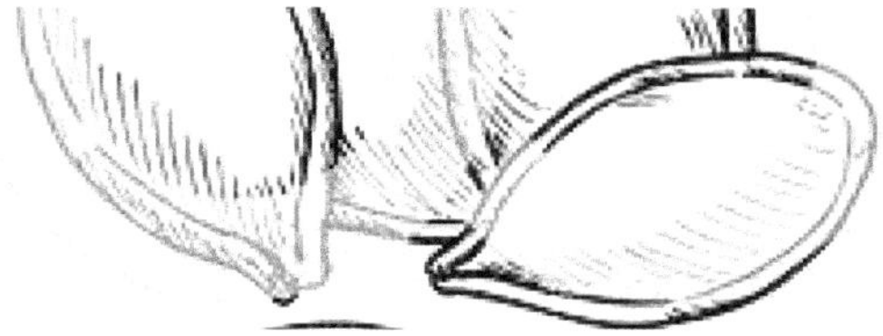

Serves: many

Prep Time: 25 min

Cook Time: 20 min

Ingredients

2 cups of pumpkin seed

1 qt water

2 tbsp salt for water

1 tsp salt for seed mix

1 tbsp margarine melted

1 tsp cracked organic pepper

1 tsp cayenne pepper (optional)

2 tsp hot pepper sauce (optional)

1 tsp paprika

Instructions

1: Preheat oven to 250F

2: Discard any cut seeds, remove stringy fibres from seeds

3: In a medium pot, combine water and salt. Bring to a boil.

4: Add seeds and boil for 10 minutes. Drain and dry.

5: Place seeds in a bowl and combine with melted vegan margarine and pepper, paprika, cayenne, hot sauce and salt.

6: Spread on a baking sheet, turn seeds every 10 minutes, bake for 30 minutes or until crisp and brown.

7: Enjoy!

Now you know what to do with all those pumpkin seeds in the fall, just eat and enjoy!

Kale Chips

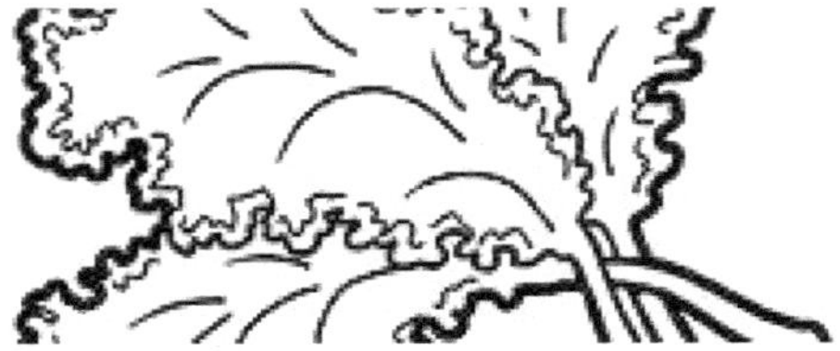

Serves: 2 to 4

Prep Time: 10 min

Cook Time: 15 min

Instructions

1. Preheat oven to 350F. Separate kale leaves and wash thoroughly and dry. Cut each leaf into quarters. In a large bowl mix olive oil, nutritional yeast, black pepper and garlic powder (and cayenne pepper if you want to spice it up).
2. Toss the kale in the mixture making sure each piece is completely coated. Once coated place kale leaves on a baking sheet in single layers.
3. Bake for 15 to 20 minutes turning over occasionally. At 15 minutes check if crisp enough.
4. Remove from oven when crispy but before edges start to char.
5. Let cool and enjoy!

Ingredients

1 large head of kale

1 tbsp olive oil

1/4 cup nutritional yeast

1 tsp black pepper

1/2 tsp garlic powder

1/2 tsp cayenne (optional)

Good Old Popped Corn

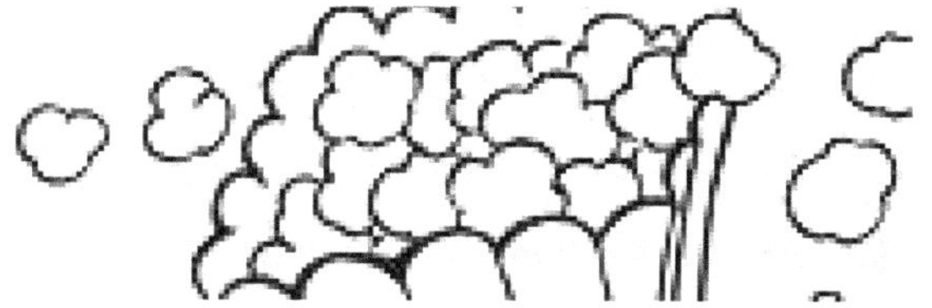

Serves: many

Prep Time: 2 min

Cook Time: 5 min

Ingredients

1 cup organic popcorn kernels

2 tbsp olive oil

1 tsp salt

1 tbsp nutritional yeast

Instructions

1. Heat on medium high in a big saucepan on stove top with olive oil.
2. When oil is hot, pour in kernels. When kernels are coated with oil cover with lid.
3. Move pan on surface back and forth to prevent kernels from burning.
4. Occasionally lift lid slightly, enough to let out some steam.
5. When popping starts to become occasional, take off heat.
6. Pour beautiful corn into big bowl and salt and nutritional yeast and mix up.

Gourmet Popcorn

Try experimenting with your favourite sauces and spices in your popcorn.

- Hot sauce
- Rosemary
- Cinnamon and brown sugar
- Garlic and onion powder
- Cayenne and paprika

Perfect Pretzel

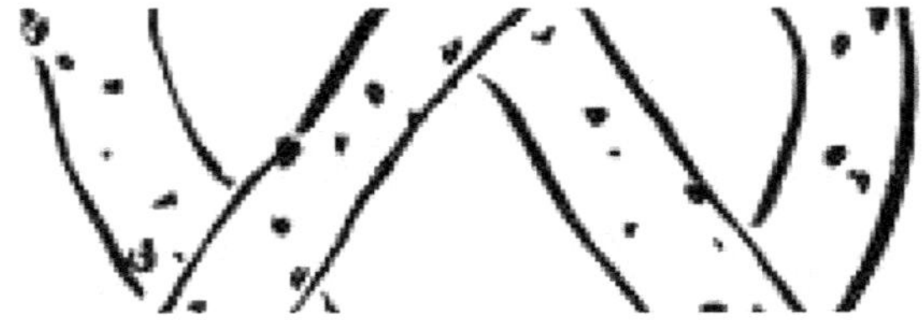

Serves: 6+

Prep Time: 35 min

Cook Time: 15 min

Instructions

1. In a bowl add sugar and yeast to water. Stir gently to incorporate and let sit for 10 minutes.
2. After 10 minutes, add melted butter and stir.
3. Slowly start to incorporate flour using a stand mixer or mixing by hand with a spatula. Continue adding flour and mixing until you have achieved a firm dough. Dough should be firm but not sticky, yet not too dry where it can be easily pulled apart. Place dough in a large mixing bowl and drizzle 1 tsp of oil over dough. Use hands to rub over the surface of the dough. Cover the bowl with a damp towel and let sit for 20 minutes.
4. In the meantime start bringing 10 cups of water to a boil. Have baking soda ready to go. Preheat oven to 400°.
5. After the dough has rested for 20 minutes knead for 5 minutes on a floured surface. Using a knife or a cutter, divide the dough into 12 equal pieces.
6. Roll each individual piece out to a rope approximately 18" long. Form the rope into a large "U" shape. Take the ends and twist twice. Take the two arms and pull them to the bottom of the circle to form the pretzel shape.
7. When all 12 pretzels have been formed, its time for the soda bath. **Slowly** add the baking soda to the boiling water (if added too fast it will boil over). Drop one pretzel into the boiling soda bath at a time for 30 seconds, flipping the pretzel after 15 seconds. Remove pretzel from the soda bath and place on a parchment paper lined baking sheet. Repeat this process until all pretzels have been boiled.
8. Brush the top of each pretzel with melted vegan margarine and sprinkle course sea salt (and chopped rosemary if desired) over top of each pretzel.
9. Bake for 15-18 minutes until golden brown. Remove from oven and serve warm.
10. Enjoy!

Ingredients

4 cups of all purpose or baking flour

1 1/2 tbsp melted vegan margarine

1 1/2 tsp fine sea salt

1 tbsp sugar (brown is best)

2 1/4 tsp or 1 pack of active dry yeast

1 1/2 cups of warm water

Course sea salt for topping

2 tbsp chopped rosemary for topping (optional)

2 tbsp melted vegan butter for topping

Baking Soda Bath

10 cups of water

3/4 cups of baking soda

Furry Friend Treats

Friend *noun*— An associate you know well and regard with affection and trust. Our “pets”.

1: Natural Doggie Treats

2: Good Dog Treats

3: Grain –Free Dog Treats

Natural Doggie Treats

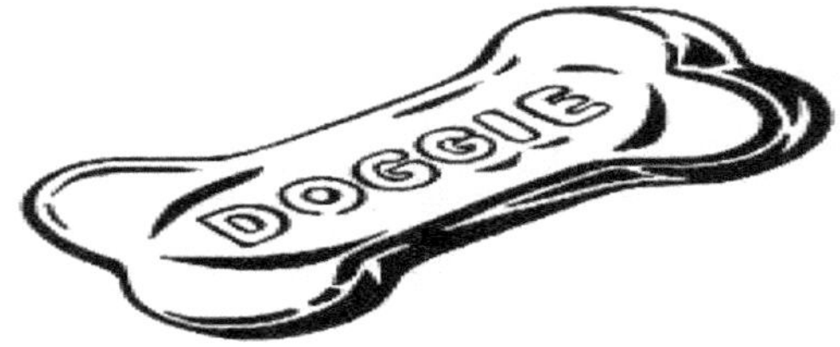

Serves: many dogs

Prep Time: 25 min

Cook Time: 15 min

Instructions

1. Mix dry ingredients.
2. Add approximately 3 cups water.
3. Knead into a pliable dough.
4. Roll out to 1/8" thickness. Cut into desired shapes.
5. Bake for 10-15 minutes at 350°F.

   Note: After turning off oven, leave biscuits in the oven overnight or for an 8-hour period so they become hard and crunchy.

   Your loyal little friends will enjoy!

Nutritional Yeast for Dogs

Nutritional yeast is a yellow flakey inactive yeast not the same brewer's yeast. Nutritional yeast is high in B-12 and a rich source of amino acids also containing protein, zinc and folic acid. Nutritional yeast contains no whey or animal products and is a low fat food.

Ingredients

9 cups spelt flour (buckwheat is a good flour for our babies too)

1 cup nutritional yeast

1 tbsp sea salt

1 tbsp garlic powder

3 cups spring water

Good Dog Cookie

Serves: many

Prep Time: 25 min

Cook Time: 30 min

Instructions

1. Peel your bananas and mash them with the peanut butter until smooth. Mix in flour until thoroughly mixed.
2. With hands form a solid ball of dough. Chill the dough for 20 minutes.
3. Remove the dough from the fridge and place on parchment paper or on a well floured counter. Preheat to 325 F.
4. Roll out the dough to a 1/2" thickness. Using your cookie cutter, cut out shapes as desired.
5. Transfer your cookies to a parchment lined baking sheet. Poke fork into each cookie twice to allow steam to escape.
6. Bake for 30 minutes. Remove and let completely cool

FYI

Give your fur-baby a good healthy treat and you can eat them too :)

Ingredients

1 cup oat or rice flour

2 or 3 ripe bananas, mashed

1/4 cup natural peanut butter

Grain-Free Dog Treat

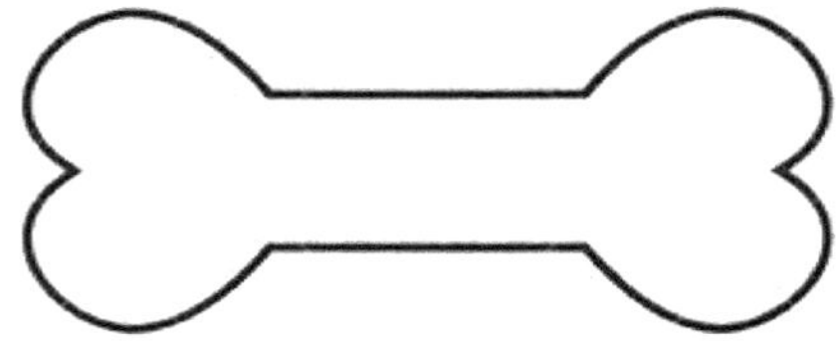

Serves: many

Prep Time: 25 min

Cook Time: 30 min

Ingredients

1 ½ cups chickpea flour

1/2 cup natural peanut butter

1/2 cup pumpkin puree

Instructions

1. In a large bowl, combine the chickpea flour, pumpkin puree , and peanut butter. knead by hand until it forms a dough ball. If the dough feels very sticky, keep adding chickpea flour until the dough is smooth and not sticky.
2. Cover it in plastic wrap and keep it in the fridge for 1 hour. This will make the dough stiffer and easier to cut shapes out of.
3. Line a cookie sheet or baking pan with parchment paper.
4. Sprinkle chickpea flour on counter and dust the rolling pin as well.
5. Sprinkle chickpea flour on the dough until there is a light coating on it, then roll out the dough to 1 inch thickness.
6. Use a cookie cutter and cut out shapes in the dough. It is crucial to dip the cookie cutter in the chickpea flour in between each cooking cutting to prevent the dough from sticking to it. If you don't have a cookie cutter, you can cut them into squares or rectangles with a knife.
7. Place on a parchment paper lined cookie sheet put in oven at 350F for 30 minutes.
8. Let cool and store in air-tight container.

References

References— Where facts and information came from other than our memory :)

References

1: The Prescription For Natural Healing—Phyllis A. Balch CNC

2: Encyclopedia Of Natural Healing—Siegfried Gursche

3: www.healthline.com

4: www.pbs.com

5: Kimberly's mom

6: Alistair's mom

Acknowledgments

Our cookery book has been inspired from the many friends, family and customers at our Alcona Beach Health Shoppe that crave a healthier lifestyle and have the need for a daily menu. For you we are very thankful.

Thank you to the contributors of some of our recipes. Mom-G, you have perfected the culinary capabilities of tofu! Mommy, your many ongoing delicious vegan meals are sublime!!

To all the organic farmers, carry on! Everyone is headed in your direction. The more we buy organic, the more the grocery stores must supply it. Keep buying organic!

Thank you to all the people all over the world that have dedicated their lives or make it part of their lives to protect animals. Thank you to PETA, you are the leader. We are both very proud to be part of your committed success.

To everyone who knows the ridicule of others who are not “woke” to the healthy alkaline lifestyle , just pray that they will one day want to have good health too. Lead by example. HEALTH IS THE ONLY WEALTH THAT MATTERS!

Live healthy and happily always,

Kimberly and Alistair

HEALTHY AND INFORMATIVE ALKALINE VEGAN COOKERY BOOK

He who has health, has hope; and he who has hope, has everything - Thomas Carlyle

Take care of your body. It's the only place you have to live - Jim Rohn

From the bitterness of disease man learns the sweetness of health - Catalan Proverb

No disease that can be treated by diet should be treated with any other means - Maimonides

Your body is a temple, but only if you treat it as one - *Astrid Alauda*

So many people spend their health gaining wealth, and then have to spend their wealth to regain their health - A J Reb Materi

It is health that is the real wealth and not pieces of gold and silver - Mahatma Gandhi

To keep the body in good health is a duty, otherwise we shall not be able to keep our mind strong and clear - Buddha

Each patient carries his own doctor inside him - Albert Schweitzer

The doctor of the future will be oneself - Thomas Edison

If you don't take care of this the most magnificent machine that you will ever be given...where are you going to live? - Karyn Calabrese

LET FOOD BE THY MEDICINE AND MEDICINE BE THY FOOD - HIPPOCRATES

When health is absent, wisdom cannot reveal itself, art cannot manifest, strength cannot fight, wealth becomes useless, and intelligence cannot be applied - Herophilus

Without health life is not life - Andy Rickford

A healthy outside starts from the inside - Robert Urich

The first wealth is health - Ralph Waldo Emerson

FriesenPress

One Printers Way
Altona, MB R0G 0B0
Canada

www.friesenpress.com

First Edition — 2021

ISBN
978-1-03-911402-9 (Hardcover)
978-1-03-911401-2 (Paperback)
978-1-03-911403-6 (eBook)

1. COOKING, VEGETARIAN & VEGAN

Distributed to the trade by The Ingram Book Company

www.ingramcontent.com/pod-product-compliance
Ingram Content Group UK Ltd.
Pitfield, Milton Keynes, MK11 3LW, UK
UKHW052100170925
7955UKWH00006B/287

9 781039 114012